"Lisa Schilling is a one-of-a-kind educator and fitness expert. She genuinely cares about the well-being and overall mind, body, and spiritual health of the individuals that she works with. This book, if followed with the same discipline and passion that Lisa has put into writing, will give you the results and life you have always wanted and deserved!"

Aric Bostick
International Motivational Speaker and
President of Aric Bostick Success Training, Inc.
www.aricbostick.com
Founder of The Camp of CHAMPS
www.campofchampsusa.com

"Finally, a fitness book written by a busy working mother for busy working mothers! Lisa's common-sense approach to taking control of your personal wellness makes the challenge of getting into shape feel attainable. By addressing common barriers and easy stumbling blocks, Lisa is able to make the journey toward personal wellness less daunting and seem like it is going to be a fun voyage and not a distant destination. I would recommend this book to anybody who has ever felt like there isn't enough time in the day to be healthy; it is as satisfying as it is enlightening."

Gerard J. Stanley, Jr., M.D.

"Lisa has developed an easy-to-follow reference that provides straightforward solutions with no external fluff. This book is packed with sound, practical, reader-friendly information and guidance. Her well-balanced approach to health, fitness, and wellness is a breath of fresh air in a crowded arena. This readable and practical guide is an invaluable resource for anyone who wants to develop a lifetime of wellness. Her down-to-earth style will draw you in, and the adaptable format will keep you going through to the end."

Tom Antion
Author of the best-selling presentation skills book *Wake 'em Up Business Presentations* and *Click: The Ultimate Guide to Electronic Marketing*
www.GreatInternetMarketingTraining.com

T0369256

"In this excellent book, Lisa Schilling, RN, gives us what we really need for our weight loss and fitness goals—empowerment. She realizes that we all know WHAT to do to get fit—that what we really need is the inspiration to go take the action and to stay motivated until we reach our goals. This book is packed and supplies the puzzle piece that I believe is most important for fitness success."

Dr. Clare Albright
Psychologist
www.NeurofeedbackBook.com

"There's a reason I'm known as the 'No B.S. Coach'; I dislike 'fluff' and like to get to the *difference that makes the difference*. Lisa Schilling delivers in a big way! Information is everywhere today. What is lacking, perhaps now more than ever, is compassion. As you read Lisa's book, you'll have the unique experience of getting a system that works from a woman who cares; you can feel it in her writing, and this is the *difference that makes a difference*."

Vincent Harris, M.S.
Body Language Expert and author of *The Productivity Epiphany*
www.facebook.com/l/fb0b5
www.VinceHarris.com

"Lisa Schilling is a dynamic author, wellness coach and motivational speaker who is passionate about helping individuals and organizations to experience their goals, dreams and successes. If there is one absolute truth about wellness it is that, it is never too late to begin. Whether you are just getting started or need a boost, Lisa Schilling's, *Get REAL Guide to Health and Fitness* will help you bridge the gap from where you are to where you want to be. Thank you Lisa for sharing *doable* suggestions and a plan for developing a happier and healthier life. Your knowledge and inspiration will help us all to add years to our life and life to our years!"

Dr. Tim Crowley
Motivational Speaker, Business Consultant and Workshop Trainer

The Get REAL Guide

to Health and Fitness

The Get REAL Guide
to Health and Fitness

Five Steps to Create Your Own Personal Wellness Plan

Lisa Schilling, RN

Trafford Publishing

Order this book online at www.trafford.com
or email orders@trafford.com

Most Trafford titles are also available at major online book retailers.

Exercise Photographs and Cover Photograph: Renea Lynch
Interior Design: Kimberly Martin
Edited: Kathy Carter
Printed in the United States of America.

ISBN: 978-1-4269-3445-2 (sc)
ISBN: 978-1-4269-3446-9 (dj)

Library of Congress Control Number:2010908669

Our mission is to efficiently provide the world's finest, most comprehensive book publishing service, enabling every author to experience success. To find out how to publish your book, your way, and have it available worldwide, visit us online at www.trafford.com

Trafford rev. 07/06/2010

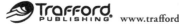 www.trafford.com

North America & international
toll-free: 1 888 232 4444 (USA & Canada)
phone: 250 383 6864 ♦ fax: 812 355 4082

My passion lies not only in showing people *what* to do to be healthier, but in helping people discover a *reason* to *want* to, and *motivation* to continue to.

Acknowledgments

This guide is dedicated to my family, friends, and the ladies of "First Place."

To my wonderful husband Shawn, who put up with me and my crazy time demands and supported all of my endeavors, even when they seemed far-fetched.

To my three boys, Cole, Sam, and Luke, who did their best to remind me what's really important in life.

To my close family members, who have always supported and encouraged me along my own personal journey.

To my friends, especially to Vicki Wheeler for her input and advice that helped this guide come together. A special thanks to Barbara Gaines for her expert guidance concerning my text presentation and Angela Dugan for her formatting expertise. Also, Renea Lynch at Look At Me Photography, for her wonderful photos and cover shot.

To the ladies of my "First Place" groups and my exercise class gals—I learned as much from you all as you ever learned from me.

To the staff at Trenton R-9, especially Lynn Daniels, Shirley King, and Sabra Ferguson, for believing in me and letting me try my concepts out on them.

To the community leaders of Trenton who continue to support me, from my years attending school through my years of working there.

To all my mentors who have influenced me to become the person I am, especially (the late) Steve Orwig and Sharon Wilken. Others include Paul and Lelar Corbett, Taryn Corbett Kinney, Steve Maxey, Kay Lea, Pat Rinehart, and Aimee Cohen. There have been many others along the way. They taught me to take good advice and not listen when people said I could not achieve something. I hope to give back in the same way I was given. I have been blessed in this life, in order to be a blessing to others, through the power of Jesus Christ who is the basis of all good things.

Table of Contents

PREFACE

A personal note from the author…

My main motivation for creating this guide was a desire to share with others what I have found personally beneficial, as well as techniques that have been helpful when working with others. This is meant to be a *comprehensive* guide. It is designed to help a diverse group of people map their *own* plan and begin a journey toward better health and fitness. I researched and studied many of the vast resources available and summarized the pertinent points, putting them in one spot.

My goal was to sort through the mountain of information and give people who struggle in this area a place to start. It was important for me to create a flexible outline that could be used by people in various circumstances. I wanted it to take into consideration the unique situations and preferences of each reader. Many of my concepts focus on your mental approach. I believe that by changing how you think about food and exercise, you can start to evaluate what drives you and what stops you in your tracks. This knowledge can be used to create a lifestyle that will allow you to *naturally* achieve your heartfelt goals.

Disclaimer: I am a registered nurse and certified personal trainer through AFAA (Aerobics and Fitness Association of America). I am neither a dietitian nor a physician. The content of this guide is a compilation of information and is based on my personal studies, observations, and findings. I am a nurse, fitness director, and wellness coach helping people from all walks of life improve their overall wellness, fitness, and health.

Never attempt a fitness routine without consulting a physician, especially if you have health issues that could be exacerbated with exercise or dietary changes. The author is not liable for any injuries or problems incurred as a result of information offered in this guide. Remember: when in doubt, check it out. You should always make choices that are in your own best interest. Knowledge is power!

Get REAL Note: This material is not to be reproduced for anyone other than the person purchasing this guide. Please do not reproduce and distribute this material. Any page may be reproduced for the *personal use* of the user.

INTRODUCTION

Get REAL Mission

As a result of this guide, you will:

1. Gain a new understanding about your relationship with food and the REAL (Realistic Expectations About Life) reasons you struggle with weight or other wellness issues.

2. Gain a greater understanding of the dynamics of exercise and healthy nutrition (*what* to do, *how* to do it, *what* happens to you when you do, *why* it works, *why* sporadic attempts often fail, and *why* you need to make it part of your everyday life).

3. Understand and explore the mental aspect of health, wellness, and fitness. This is often the most important of all. Those who have struggled with these issues for many years need this the most. When your head and heart are into it, you will succeed!

4. Be able to use the information presented to construct your own Personal Wellness Plan.

So now it's time to get on board with Get REAL thinking and learn how to construct your plan. Along this journey I will introduce you to twenty Get REAL Concepts and several Get REAL five-step breakdowns. You will also come across Get REAL Notes, Points, Ideas, Tips, and Bottom Lines. You will use all of these to help shape your plan. The outline for creation of a solid Personal Wellness Plan is laid out for you.

The complicated part is putting the wheels in motion, determining your choices, and actually doing what you have determined will work for you. Remember . . .

> **Any plan is only as good as your willingness to do it!**

The Five Get REAL Steps for Creating Your Own Personal Wellness Plan

1. **Line up your thinking!** Honestly evaluate your schedule and assess personal needs. Determine what you want to achieve and what you'll get from it. Your mental preparation is essential for all lifestyle improvement.

Rationale: To succeed, you must first understand what you hope to get from new behaviors and what is realistic for you personally.

2. **Create a healthy outline.** To shape your lifestyle, you must make decisions that will become the outline for your daily choices. This forms accountability and gives you direction. You must block off time each day for exertion and for recovery. Honor this cycle by scheduling equal recovery time for the exertion activities you are adding.

Rationale: In order to reach your goals, you must outline what you want and how you plan to get it. Without this basic step, your efforts will be random and unfruitful. Seek to create balance in your daily activities. Setting your direction and creating accountability gives you direct control over your outcome.

3. **Select a nutrition strategy.** Choose a plan that fits you and your lifestyle (use the results of #1). This is a way of thinking about *food*, not a strict *diet*. You will determine a way of eating that meets your needs and that will help you meet your goals. When you eat following *your* guidelines, you will see favorable outcomes. If you struggle with making good choices, being accountable to someone can help.

Rationale: Eating purposefully, with clear and flexible guidelines, will enable you to reach your goals without going crazy. Always plan

5

ahead—purposeful eating to produce a result will provide structure and reduce confusion over what and when to eat. Proper planning ensures you have what it takes to stay on track.

4. **Select an exercise option.** Chose an option that fits your needs, and create a workable and flexible exercise incorporation plan. Make yourself accountable for daily movement, even if it is only five to ten minutes. Purposefully plan time for exercise by building it into your daily Fitness Plan. Check in with someone regularly if this is a difficult step.

Rationale: Exercise does more than condition the body. It releases endorphins in the brain that elevate mood and produce feelings of well-being. As you age, strengthening bones and muscle becomes invaluable. Exercise can improve your overall quality of life.

5. **Develop your lifetime wellness lifestyle.** Wellness is a way of life. It will permeate every choice you make. Throughout this guide, you will be taught healthy behaviors and how to incorporate them into daily life. For health and wellness to be lifelong, you must plan on making them a part of your regular lifestyle.

Rationale: By gradually learning and implementing healthy behaviors, you can develop a lifestyle that promotes and maintains wellness. Random or short-term attempts will not affect the permanent changes that you seek. Cultivate your lifetime wellness and it will blossom into an enjoyable, healthy lifestyle.

Be accountable to your plan. Use an accountability group or partner if you have trouble maintaining your focus. Start slow and gradually build up to your goal by using the 10 percent rule: gradually increase your efforts by only 10 percent at a time instead of making vast changes that cannot be maintained in the long term. As you read the upcoming chapters, consider the concepts offered. Each person will use the information in personally unique ways. Feel free to jot notes in the margins, highlight thoughts that speak to you, or make separate notes. This is a guide, a reference booklet. You may utilize it in any way that meets your needs. It is interactive, so fill in the blanks to shape your Personal Wellness Plan. The chapters to come give detailed information on specific health and wellness techniques to choose from.

Get REAL Note: Remember to always enjoy the journey! It is not all about *reaching* your goals; it is about *living* them every day. So get started and make it fun.

PART I

LINE UP YOUR THINKING

CHAPTER 1

It's Time to Get REAL!

Good for you! The fact that you opened this guide means that you are ready to figure out how to make some positive changes in your lifestyle—realistic changes that will last for a lifetime. Beware—if you are thinking of putting this book down or starting to just thumb through it—STOP! There are some REAL reasons that got you to your current health and fitness level. How did I know that you were considering this? I have been there.

I was always looking for the quick fix. I studied, researched, and looked into every theory that came down the pike. From trial and error, I have learned some valuable lessons. Going from a young pageant queen to an older, overweight wife and mother of three boys has given me some unique perspectives. I have faced the ebb and flow of yo-yo diets and weight cycling. And the journey brought me to this conclusion: "There must be a better way to do things!" So I embarked on a mission of health and fitness education for myself, our school, and our community. I started by realizing that my own health and fitness habits had declined and in many areas had become nonexistent.

My life had evolved into what many people find as they develop multiple responsibilities—too *busy*, too *tired*, and too *overwhelmed* to schedule time for myself and my own health. I saw it as another "thing" on my list of things I needed to do. Have you ever been there? I found out that many people *are* there. I was not alone in my negative health and fitness thinking. But as a nurse, wellness coach, and former pageant

11

winner, it seemed worse for me to think this way. In short, I knew better. But in this, I discovered my first . . .

> **Get REAL Point:**   Just because you know the right things to do, does not mean you will choose to do them.

In this dilemma, my philosophy was born. We need to Get REAL! Life was easier to maintain before having a husband, three boys, a household, and a full-time job. What a surprise! But as my life changed, I lost the ability to maintain my previous health and fitness standards. Unfortunately, "experts" in this industry only tell people the restrictive, highest standards that you would follow if you had all the time, motivation, and resources to work on achieving optimum health. But most people live in the "REAL world," and that is not something they are able to commit to for the long haul. Many start—they try to follow these rigid standards— then ultimately give up due to how difficult they are to maintain.

This crazy setup forces people into "all-or-nothing" patterns, the results of which are yo-yo diets and weight cycling. What was intended to improve people's health is now the cause of chronic poor health and decreased fitness. So, what could I do about this? I discovered a purpose—to find out how to get back what I once had, in the new lifestyle I currently have. By helping myself, I knew I would be able to help others who have found themselves in similar positions. That is my passionate purpose for creating this guide.

> **Get REAL Note:**   The big "ah-hah moment" came when I realized that there needed to be a more *obtainable entry point* into health and fitness improvement.

I found that starting small, at less than what "experts" say is optimal, made it easier to stick to my plan and actually see improvement. Seems too simple, I know—but confidence gained from sticking with something and having success propels you to add more healthy habits. Small changes, consistently and slowly done, actually work!

This goes against the severe all-or-nothing mentality that I fight daily. I have lost and gained over thirty pounds at a time. It is a struggle I will always have. But I have a choice. I have learned how to gradually change my thinking and my habits. I now understand the value of appreciating my situation and changing as my needs change. I must fight to avoid those all-or-nothing patterns—it is a daily choice. You have a choice too. Because of thought shifting, reframing, and purposeful living, you have the ability to greatly improve your fitness and total wellness, not to mention increase personal fulfillment.

If this type of planning worked for me, I knew it could help others. This spurred me to coordinate the Great Green Hills Weight Loss Challenge. There were 250 participants the first year and 400 participants the next year. It became clear that many people were looking for ways to get healthier and for something to motivate and keep them on track. I saw a need to help people from different backgrounds and fitness levels find a way to get healthier and stay healthy, all the while living their normal REAL life.

The Internet, bookstores, and TV are full of information about what to do and how to do it. That is the problem—information overload! Who has time to sort through that pile of information? It can be so overwhelming that some people give up before they even start. After a while, people stop listening to the advice available. It becomes like the teacher in the Peanuts cartoons: "wah, wah, wah." They tune it out because they are simply not motivated enough to deal with it. I have come to understand that the phrase "I don't have time" really means "I just don't want to *that* badly." Because the truth is, you will figure out a way to do the things you really want to do.

> **Get REAL Note:** The roadblock to helping more people achieve better health is unlocking their motivation. There needs to be less talk about *what* to do and more time spent helping people figure out a tangible reason to *want* to do it. We must also help to uncover a lasting motivation that will *keep* them doing it.

It is imperative that you discover what will work for you, not copy what someone else has done. This requires some self-discovery. You will use what you learn about yourself to formulate your own Personal Wellness Plan. I will walk you through the basic steps. Each step is a rung on the ladder of your life. You step up one rung at a time until you reach your goal. You don't jump from the bottom to the top in one massive leap (crash scenario). *This is a process.*

You did not suddenly wake up one morning in your current shape. It has evolved from comfortable patterns. This guide is designed to address what got you here in the first place. You will use that information to begin mapping out your own journey forward. Living a healthy lifestyle needs to become something you enjoy, look forward to, and live on a daily basis! Not a short-term fix, something to dread, or a painful sacrifice. You have time—use it!

Living healthy, happy, and fit always requires something of you. Creating your own Personal Wellness Plan is good place to start. But as noted earlier, any plan is only as good as your willingness to actually do it regularly. You will only get from your efforts what you put into them. Think—no investment, no return! This investment will reap big dividends, empowering you to *enjoy* your crazy, busy, and unique life.

Get REAL Note: Embrace life—no more dieting and restricting, no more failure, and no more guilt.

Guilt serves as a self-imposed prison for people with good intentions to check themselves into. This happens when you fail to meet the standards you have set for yourself. Well-meaning people—forgetting they are human—hold themselves back when they check into the "prison of guilt." Guilt sends you rushing back to the coping behaviors that got you where you are in the first place. Do not let guilt or shame make you a prisoner.

This personal acceptance is another key to unlock your potential, and it allows you the freedom to explore who you were meant to be, to find your passionate purpose. You hold this key too. Choose to turn it and set yourself free from the *guilt-dread-inaction* cycle. Remember that how and what you think—your internal dialogue—will impact your overall success.

Successful people do not suffer from the catch-22 of guilt leading to lack of progress. They don't let what they *should have done* hold them back. To succeed, you must learn to accept that you are human and you will make choices that, in hindsight, you will wish you could change. When you begin to accept that you are okay—even better than okay— just as you are, you will empower yourself to succeed at making any changes that you choose.

Get REAL Tip: Don't think "diet," think "plan." It is time to stop dieting and start planning!

There is not one plan that is perfect for everyone. This book puts *you* in the driver's seat. It gives you all the information you need to create a REAL plan that will work for *you*. I identified the main reasons I have found that REAL people struggle, and I addressed those issues. I wanted to take the knowledge I have gained through research, trial and error, and working with everyday people to compile an easy-to-read and easy-to-understand guide.

I have used that information, plus what I give to my personal training clients, to develop this guide. I realized that REAL people need an encouraging resource—one that is short, easy to understand, basic, and comprehensive. That is what I have set out to do. If you choose to follow this guide, you will be able to customize your own unique plan. A *plan* for life—an enjoyable REAL life!

> **Get REAL Bottom Line:** Living a healthy lifestyle involves having a *plan* and *living purposefully.*

CHAPTER 2

Unlocking Your Motivational Code

Most people know that to lose weight and be healthier, they need to eat better and exercise more. The problem is they have not unlocked a way to do this while living their normal, REAL life. People are unique; each holds a unique sequence or code that unlocks his or her personal motivation to succeed. The goal then becomes to find out that code and to put it in the right sequence that unlocks that person's unique motivators.

> **Get REAL Point:** You hold the "combination" to unlock your success. Now is the time to choose whether you will discover it.

So in true Get REAL fashion, let's be honest. Whatever your current level of health and wellness, it is a direct result of your personal habits practiced over time. If your situation is less than desirable, then you need to accept accountability for it. No more excuses, no more blaming and complaining! Note that I am not talking about people with chronic disease or illness that was unpreventable. I am talking to those of you, like myself, who often choose the path of least resistance when it comes to lifestyle choices.

Whatever habit you keep, there is a payoff (motivation) for keeping it, or you simply wouldn't continue it. The only way to change this pattern is to find a new payoff (motivator) for the behaviors you want to cultivate. Whatever you decide, take responsibility for the choice.

Is this starting to click now? I can almost hear the tumblers turning as you start to "unlock" your thinking.

If you experience the same "comfort glaze" I get when I come home and sit down—do a reality check! The chances of you jumping up and starting that exercise routine or enjoying a different way of eating are slim if you are not altering your routine—not only altering your routine, but also having a meaningful *purpose* to do so. If you do not, the "comfort glaze" will call to you and lull you into "I'll start tomorrow" thinking.

Motivation can be external or internal. What works for one person may have no effect on another. We have seen people be motivated by the goal of winning a prize, by the desire to avoid embarrassment by having results made public, or by the accountability of reporting to someone. Just knowing you "need to do it" does not motivate most people enough to make changes.

Your challenge is to discover an external motivator to make achieving your goal worthwhile and then to alter your routine specifically to accommodate the achievement of your goal. Focus on what achieving your goal will do for you, not on what you "should" be doing. If you make the payoff big enough, you will put in the extra effort to get it done. Here is a five-step breakdown to help you get started.

The Five Get REAL Steps to Jump-Start Your Goal!

- Set a realistic goal.
- Create a worthy payoff.
- Set up accountability.
- Alter your routine to fit in the changes.
- Finally—stick to it!

Many people include the goal of weight loss on their list of reasons to start a wellness program. This is a valid reason; however, it tends to not be a strong enough motivator unless combined with other, more pressing factors. This has to do with personal comfort levels. Every behavior or habit that is repeated must have that payoff. For some, the payoff is simply comfort or pleasure. For others, the payoff may be feedback from peers or loved ones.

Most of the negative health habits you keep are based in comfort. You do what you feel like doing and what is most convenient, especially when you lack multiple motivators to keep you accountable. Make no mistake, there is comfort in the familiar, and to change that will take some hearty motivation and discipline.

Three-Phase Get REAL Weight Loss

Successful weight loss is best achieved in three phases. When you decide, "This is it, I am done! I am going to change my weight and my habits," then you are ready to start the Three-Phase Get REAL Weight Loss plan.

Get REAL Note: To reach the goal of weight loss, you must first clearly decide why losing weight is more important than continuing the comfort of your regular habits.

Phase I Weight Loss involves developing an exercise introduction plan. It can take from four to eight weeks to establish this phase. It is a way of easing you into a new routine. The reasons are twofold. First, you want to avoid burning out, and second, you want to avoid injury. Starting slow and gradually building your exercise routine by 10 percent weekly is the smartest way to lose weight and keep it off. Is it the fastest? No, but it has the greatest probability of becoming a lifelong change.

When you create a gradual progression of exercise, you will build upon each success until you have comfortably made exercise a part of your lifestyle. This is very important! If exercise does not become part of your lifestyle, you will be doomed to repeat your past failures. When treated like a temporary solution, exercise serves as nothing more than a Band-Aid on a large wound that needs stitches.

> **Get REAL Point:** Building a program that makes exercise a part of your regular lifestyle is paramount to maintaining lifelong health and weight loss.

Phase II Weight Loss involves developing a peak weight loss routine. In this phase, you have established a solid exercise routine and have been committed to sticking with it. Now it is time to ramp up your efforts. This means committing more time to cardio exercise in your target heart rate. You will need to increase the number of days you exercise, the number of minutes, and the intensity. Sound tough? It is—if weight loss were easy, we would all be thin. You will also need to begin increasing the amount of weight you use during resistance training. It becomes even more important to keep challenging your muscles to work harder for you. A minimum of two full-body workouts per week will be necessary.

This targeted peak routine will need to continue until you meet your goal. Ouch!—I know that seems tough, but it is time to take off the rose-colored glasses. If you want *Biggest Loser*-type results, then you will need to put in *Biggest Loser*-type efforts. This goes back to the question "How bad do you want this?" If the motivation to work hard is not there, you may want to save yourself the aggravation—or better yet, just uncover your personal motivator and get to it!

Phase III Weight Loss is maintenance. Once you achieve your goal, you will have to continue your lifetime wellness plan to maintain it. The good news is that you can scale back from the Phase II peak stage. The general recommendation for health is 120 minutes per week of physical exercise. That could be thirty minutes, four times a week. Most people find that to be very achievable. The trick is making exercise a regular and nonnegotiable part of your lifestyle. Phase III is a lifetime *lifestyle* of fitness. For weight loss and good health to be lifelong, exercise and eating purposefully needs to become "just something you do."

Some people argue that losing weight is easier for men than women. Learning how people differ in the area of weight loss can be motivating to those who have become discouraged by discrepancies. I will briefly explain some of these issues in an attempt to show that they can be overcome with proper wellness strategies. Part of unlocking your motivation is learning about the processes that you are engaged in. This step will empower you to make informed choices as they are presented to you.

> **Get REAL Note:** There is a basic equation for the balance of energy. It shows that energy in (calories) minus energy out (metabolism and activity) equals body weight.

From the perspective of energy balance and the ability to lose weight, there are several physiological ways that people differ. One issue is size. The larger you are, the more calories your body burns at rest and during activity. This is due to moving a greater mass through space.

Another difference is the fat-to-muscle ratio. A woman's natural body composition has a greater fat percentage and less lean muscle than a man's. This is due to the reproductive organs and the essential fat needed for childbearing. Men require only 3 percent essential body fat, whereas women require a whopping 12 percent.

Testosterone levels are another issue. This hormone enhances the building of lean muscle mass. Women possess only a fraction of the testosterone of men. As a result, men have twenty to thirty times the muscle-building potential of women. The more muscle mass you possess, the greater rate of calorie burn you will have.

One pound of muscle can burn between thirty-five and fifty calories per day. So just one pound of muscle can help you burn 5.2 pounds in a year. Five pounds of muscle would burn twenty-six pounds. Studies show that by adding muscle mass, you can raise your metabolic rate anywhere from 7 to 15 percent. This results from the breakdown and repair of muscle tissue caused by the stress of resistance training.

> **Get REAL Point:**   Adding lean muscle will raise your metabolism. This enables you to eat more and still lose weight.

Another issue is osteoporosis or bone loss. This occurs as both men and women age. The problem is that women start their lives with less bone mass than men, causing a greater percentage of loss. Excessive dieting, calcium deficiencies, and menopause simply add to this problem. With menopause comes a whole range of issues. It is a time of vast hormonal changes for women. Age-related bone loss is accelerated for women during the first five to seven years after menopause. During this time, they can lose as much as 20 percent of their bone mass. Weight-bearing exercise can stop and often reverse this age-related bone loss.

Aging also causes an accelerated loss of lean muscle tissue. The average person, man or woman, will lose between one-half and seven-tenths of a pound of muscle yearly. But as women approach menopause, that amount of muscle loss almost doubles! This will account for a large drop in metabolism and daily calorie burning. As estrogen diminishes, women can also experience a compositional shift to weight storage around the abdominal area.

Besides menopause, women deal with hormonal fluctuations during their monthly cycle and throughout their childbearing years. Issues such as bloating, cravings, emotional instability, low energy, irritability, and sleep problems can lead to bouts of depression and feelings of anxiety. These serious problems can cause a greater release of cortisol, a stress hormone, which can trigger fat storage. This instability of hormones makes weight loss and motivation for exercise more difficult. Although this sounds very disheartening—do not despair. There is hope! A lifestyle change, including weight-bearing exercise, can help tip the scales back in your favor.

Get REAL Note: By starting a program of good nutrition, cardiopulmonary exercise, and progressive weight training, the negative side effects of aging can be halted and often reversed.

Total wellness is like a four-legged stool. It consists of resistance training, cardiopulmonary exercise, nutrition, and mental-emotional health. Kick one of the legs out from under the stool and you know what will happen. The same will happen to your efforts if you do not incorporate all four areas into your lifetime wellness plan. These areas will be detailed in the chapters to come. They will all be approached from a factual but realistic perspective.

I believe knowledge is power. By learning about how your body works, your chances of developing lasting motivation are enhanced.

Armed with this knowledge and realistic strategies, you can begin to create healthier habits.

This guide aims to have you forget everything you ever *thought* you knew about preservation of health and fitness. Often, deeply held perceptions keep people from finding REAL solutions to overcome their past issues. Old thinking will hold you in bondage to feelings of dread and inadequacy. Traditional teaching will leave you overwhelmed and unequipped to find success in your uniquely busy REAL life.

This book is not about traditional standard recommendations. That kind of advice does not consider each person holistically and individually—it promotes what someone could do in the vacuum of an ideal situation. Americans keep growing larger and unhealthier because that kind of traditional advice is not realistic in most REAL lives. The inability to meet those high standards leads people to do nothing at all. Learning a "moderation principle" and accepting "less than perfect" is part of the solution.

Get REAL Bottom Line:	In the real world, life can be crazy. But cheer up—*you* have some control over what happens to *you*. Take what is available to you and use it to create the life you have been hoping for.

This guide is meant to rock how you think about traditional healthy living. It teaches you to enjoy the process, not just the end result. When you renew your thinking about what it takes to live healthy, you will develop increased motivation. This will enable you to actually begin enjoying your new, healthier lifestyle.

CHAPTER 3

Battlefield in the Mind: Dumping the Diet Mentality

Well, congratulations on taking the first step to a healthier you! The right frame of mind is the first battle you face when it comes to making changes. You must be *ready* to do it. It is the same for any habit you want to change. "Wanting to" is not enough. Someone telling you "you should" is not enough.

You must be ready to make the change. It requires something of you. You have to reach the point where you decide, "I have had enough! I am going to do something about this." And beyond that, there must be a REAL commitment to do what it will take to change, even when it gets difficult or inconvenient. Whew!

Why is it so hard to live a healthy lifestyle? Today you have more information on how to be healthy and more resources, yet there is more preventable illness than ever. This puzzled me at first, but after learning more I uncovered this truth: Most struggles with healthy living issues start in the mind. The brain is a complex computer. On a conscious level, you set goals based on the information you take in and know to be true. However, on a subconscious level, you have very strong but subtle programming that has been established through years of repetition and conditioning.

Whether this programming was right or wrong, true or false, the result of it is what you believe. What you believe about yourself affects every aspect of life, your chances of success, and your ability to create positive change. Programming is what you have *accepted* from the outside world or fed to yourself. It sets up your beliefs, and a chain reaction begins from that.

> **Get REAL Note:** Author Shad Helmstetter puts it like this: "In logical progression, what we believe determines our attitudes, affects our feelings, directs our behavior, and determines our success or failure."

The Programming-Results Cycle

In his book *What to Say When You Talk to Your Self*, Shad Helmstetter notes this Programming-Results Cycle:

- Programming creates beliefs.
- Beliefs create attitudes.
- Attitudes create feelings.
- Feelings determine actions.
- Actions create results.

That is how the brain works. So if you want to create healthy changes in your life, you must first address the subconscious programming you have previously accepted. How do you do that? You start by listening to your internal dialogue—you know, that little voice that keeps a running conversation in your head. The brain will introduce thoughts into your mental dialogue based on your prior programming. Often it is this subtle little detail that stands in the way of starting or maintaining healthy habits that you know in your conscious mind to be beneficial. The subconscious messages sabotage your efforts at every turn.

> **Get REAL Point:** Your mind knows only what you tell it. It believes that to be true whether it is reality or not.

If your mental dialogue is always interjecting thoughts like "I hate to exercise," "I am so tired," "I really want some junk food," and other common thought patterns, this is what your body will work to make reality. Understand that this is the root of the issue. Just as weeds have roots, so do our issues. You can mow over a weed and it may seem dealt with, for a time. But we all know that until you deal with the root, you will deal with that weed forever.

Many people deal with the weed of unhealthy habits because they never deal with the root of the problem. The root is your subconscious programming. The only way to effectively reprogram what has taken years to establish is one thought at a time. You must first recognize when those nagging negative thoughts enter your mind. Seek and destroy! You have a choice—you do not have think whatever thought falls into your head. You can say to yourself, "I am going to look at this in a new way." When those thoughts come, stop and reframe the thought. "I know that I will feel great when I get done exercising." "I will have more energy when I eat better and get a walk in." "Junk food tastes good now, but I know it leaves me hungry and wanting more. I am going to choose a snack based on what will make my body feel good for the day, not just the next few minutes."

With a little practice, *intentional thought reframing* or *thought shifting* can begin to positively affect your programming-results cycle. If you need more reinforcement, you can write common reframed thoughts on note cards and review them regularly, or even post them in frequently viewed areas. Enlist friends to prompt you to "reframe" when you speak out those negative thoughts. Together as a team, you can deal with the root of your healthy living roadblocks. Reprogramming negative thought patterns works, but just like anything, you must commit to it. I believe previous subconscious programming is what keeps most people from doing what the conscious mind wants to do.

Empower yourself and take back control of your life. The human mind is amazing. It will do anything possible that you tell it to do, if you tell it often enough and strongly enough. It unconditionally accepts what you tell it as fact and acts accordingly. Be sure you are telling it:

- I can be healthy and fit!
- I enjoy how I feel when I follow my plan.
- I deserve to be healthy and well.

Create that belief and remind yourself often. Your brain will believe it, and as a result, you will live that belief in your actions. Begin listening to what you are thinking, and actively choose to reframe any negative thoughts into statements of hope.

You do not have to accept what you have always had. But to *have* something different, you must *do* something different. People are peculiar! They truly want to continue to do what they have always done but get different results. That sounds nuts, but most people—if they were honest—would admit that this is what they would like.

It is this belief that makes the diet and fitness industry so lucrative. Companies make millions of dollars off those who want some product, pill, or plan to instantly change an undesirable situation. This product, pill, or plan is usually purchased in the hope that you can live just like you always have, but now get the desired result. This is true for all habits. It is easier to do what you have always done. People live in their comfort zone because it requires nothing of them.

No matter how busy, people often follow a general routine or set of personal behaviors. Often this is unconscious. How do you spend your free time? How do you structure your time after work or when kids get home from school? What do you do when stressed or bored? These behaviors become routines. These routines become habits.

Most often people continue the habits that are comfortable and discontinue the ones that push them beyond conscious or unconscious boundaries. That is why most New Year's resolutions are often a distant memory by February. People realize that the outcome they desire can be obtained, *in a time frame they desire*, only as a result of behaviors that are difficult to maintain daily. Note that I said, "In a time frame they desire." That really is the key.

People want what they want *now*—not later. They want to "have it now and pay later," but good health and weight loss are "pay first and get it later" deals. Not to mention that you must keep paying to maintain them. That's not a comfortable proposition for most people. They want to lose weight or improve their health *fast* so they can return to their old, comfortable patterns *faster*. This is one of the main reasons yo-yo dieters often fail and end up gaining more weight. It is the desire to *eventually* return to those comfortable patterns.

Get REAL Note: To succeed at making lifestyle changes, first change your mindset and your behaviors will follow.

It is very harmful to alter your body's natural cues this way. Been there—done that! I am someone who has struggled with weight all my life. I have never been what most would consider overweight, but I was seldom near my goal weight, and I constantly had to exercise or change my diet to maintain or lose some extra pounds.

I went through years of up and down and have real empathy for people who enjoy food and are forced to alter eating patterns to adjust body weight. The fact that I have a great deal of knowledge about fitness and nutrition does not guarantee that I will do what I know works. It is still, and always will be, a choice. "Do what is comfortable and have a less than desirable outcome" or "Do what I know works and have the outcome I desire." You face this choice too.

I am here to help you figure out how to make this time different! If you lose a large amount of weight only to gain it all back within the year, what good have you really done? I want to help people who are *ready* to make a change and give them REAL-life strategies that work in the long term. Commit to change your thinking patterns and you will see positive change in your life—great changes that you created!

Get REAL Concept 1:
Create thinking that supports what is really important in your life.

When your decisions are based on supporting your total health, you are more likely to maintain and benefit from any lifestyle changes you create. Right now, you need to create a "What Matters Most" list. This will help you evaluate the priorities in your life. As you read this guide, you will refer to the list for help in building your Personal Wellness Plan.

The people and things that matter most in my life are:

_____   _____   _____

_____   _____   _____

_____   _____   _____

_____   _____

Align each choice you make with your list. Learning to base choices on the bigger picture takes some time and practice. On this journey you will have many opportunities to try out plan-focused thinking. The fact that you're reading this information shows that you want to improve your health and fitness. This guide will provide tools that will make putting the pieces together easier and more beneficial for your long-term total health.

> **Get REAL Point:** Life can be like a jigsaw puzzle. Focus on the four corner pieces of total health. When you have them in place, the rest of the puzzle is much easier to put together.

The Four Corners of Total Health

- Nurturing your family (relationships)
- Caring for your physical body
- Making time for your mental health
- Cultivating your spiritual health

Your personality style and history of previous change attempts will influence what you need to do to make this effort a success. It is up to you to discover that new path. If you gain anything from this road map, I hope that it is a renewed perspective on behaviors that lead to long-term health and personal satisfaction. After all, life is about so much more than just numbers on a scale.

You can be thin and unhappy. Look at Hollywood to see what I mean. Many famous people have perfect bodies, lots of money, fame, and everything this world says they need to be happy, yet they are still unhappy. Many of them turn to drugs and alcohol just to cope with daily life. So be sure not to put the goal of weight loss on a pedestal. It is like anything else—just one piece in the bigger puzzle.

Get REAL Tip: Be especially mindful of what you dwell on. What you think about will manifest itself in your actions.

Fill your mind with encouraging and uplifting thoughts. There is *power* in your thoughts. Whatever you feed grows, and what you starve dies. That means whichever you feed, negative or positive thinking, that's what will grow in your life. When you stop negative thoughts before they can take root, they will not thrive. Focus on the positive! Remember, energy flows where your attention goes. What you focus on will determine your overall success. As Henry Ford stated, "Whether you think you can or you think you can't, you are right!"

Your current health and fitness attitude is a product of your thinking. When you get ready to make changes, you will—and not before. I have discovered that when I want something badly enough, I will do what it takes to obtain it. I will make sacrifices and do things that are not comfortable or easy. But if the outcome is not that important to me, then I will make excuses about why I don't want to do things or why I am not able to now.

Face reality—what is keeping you from doing what you need to do to meet your goals? Consider what's been on your mind lately. Be honest and take a Get REAL gut check! Has it been how good you are feeling about making healthy changes? How empowered you feel knowing you are getting stronger and leaner? Or is it how miserable you are because you have chosen to give up some pleasurable habits and have not replaced them? Honestly addressing the cause of your hesitations will allow you to overcome them.

Learn new ways of structuring your time that will support the gradual, moderate, and consistent changes you are trying to make. This is within your reach if you are willing to do the things you know how to do, in a moderate and maintainable way. Anything less can result in a decrease in your total health. If it's a widely accepted fact that in the long run diets do not work, then why do people continue to go on diets when they need to lose weight or become healthier?

The health, diet, and fitness industries are notorious for setting people up to fail. Why? Because they only give you "in a perfect world" scenarios. Who lives there? I sure don't! I need a realistic plan that will work in my hectic and crazy life. If it does not add to my life, I'm not going to keep up the behavior. It becomes essential to determine what adds value to any new behavior so you will keep it up.

> **Get REAL Tip:** If the horse is *dead*, dismount! Don't waste time repeating old ways that have not worked for you before.

Get REAL Concept 2:
Use *mindful thought shifting* as a tool
to combat unproductive thinking patterns.

Changing your internal dialogue, that little voice inside your head, requires you to be mindful of what you think about. You must purposefully shift from your natural thoughts to intentional, directed thinking. It is easy to fall into "lazy thinking" or "habitual thinking." This pattern of thinking requires nothing of you. It relies on old habits and the familiar.

If food is used to cope, when stress comes, your brain will naturally introduce thoughts of food to you. Why? It is familiar and comfortable. It is your brain's way of trying to help fix your problem with what you usually use. The only way you will change this pattern is to intentionally shift or reframe your thoughts to reflect your new ideas of healthy living. This will take some trial and error, but rest assured, you will get many chances to practice!

Thought shifting can be used for making positive affirmations or for trying to alter your perception of something that has been a temptation. When the brain introduces the thought of a hot fudge sundae as you pass the fast-food restaurant, you can shift that thought to something unpleasant. In your mind's eye, you can picture that sundae with a cockroach in it or imagine that someone spit on it.

Inserting that undesirable image will create an unpleasant food association. It will be harder to crave something you associate with a disgusting image. This kind of thought shifting can work with any type of food that is tempting you. This behavior can reinforce your goals and bring a greater level of success.

Being mindful of what you dwell on will make a difference in other areas as well. Stop thoughts that signal dread or make healthy behaviors seem unpleasant. Instead of allowing yourself to think, "Oh, I don't want to go for walk" or "This is so good—I am going to have seconds," insert supportive thinking: "I am at least going to walk around the block—I will feel better" or "I don't know if I can eat all of this—I am so full." This kind of intentional thinking will help you map your course in the direction you are trying to go.

Surround yourself with people and things that make living your plan easier and more fulfilling. Stack the deck in your favor. When fighting with negative internal dialogue, engage in behaviors that reinforce positive choices. Read supportive books or articles, call uplifting friends, or go walking. Continually renew and refresh positive patterns of thinking. Remember, your thoughts steer the ship. Your internal dialogue will dramatically affect the outcome of changes you are trying to make. Choose your thoughts and attitudes carefully! They will determine where and how far you go.

An attitude of gratitude can create happiness, making you feel full and complete. Research has shown that positive emotions, like gratitude and love, can enhance and strengthen the immune system, which helps the body to resist disease and recover from illness more quickly. One effect is to stimulate the dilation of blood vessels, leading to a more relaxed heart. This effect occurs due to the release of endorphins, which are the body's natural painkillers, into the bloodstream. Positive emotions and thinking can actually make you healthier!

Get REAL Tip: Change *expectations* to *expectancy.*

Purposeful thought shifting can create expectancy about new behaviors. They can become something you look forward to completing. Why? Because you realize that completing them unloads your guilt baggage over not doing them. You are now focusing on the joy of having those things done and no longer nagging yourself to do them. Procrastination is a tool we subconsciously use to put off doing the unpleasant in hopes that it will go away. However, most people never mentally let themselves off the hook, and the negative feelings procrastination creates are detrimental to progress. Recognize this trap and gain joy from doing your "most difficult to get motivated for" task first.

In his book *Eat That Frog*, Brian Tracy paraphrased Mark Twain: "If the first thing you do when you wake up in the morning is eat a live frog, then nothing worse can happen for the rest of the day!" By getting unpleasant tasks out of the way first, you will not let the dreadful anticipation of them ruin the rest of your day. You are now taking action and making a purposeful plan.

Get REAL Note: Purposeful thought shifting can be used to stop a behavior from becoming an "expectation" you must fulfill.

An unfulfilled expectation leads to dread. Dread only serves to negatively influence your internal dialogue. As was established above, internal dialogue steers your ship. The "Law of Attraction" claims that you bring to yourself what your mind dwells on. So it stands to reason that by putting your thoughts in order, you will put your steps in order, thus creating the success you desire. This is a key concept on your journey to better total health, fitness, and wellness.

Get REAL Concept 3:
Get excited about creating a new, moderate living plan.

This new way of thinking is important, because it will shape your willingness to continue the healthy habits in the long term (which is the goal). Being enthusiastic about your new way of living is part of the journey. From this point on, each choice will have more meaning and purpose. This is not a dreaded, sacrificing, procrastinating kind of plan. You create it based on your own special needs.

Realizing that you steer the ship and that you are in control of what happens will be a big part of your success. This internal control empowers you to stay on track. Realize that you don't have to do all the right things all the time in order to improve your health! Small meaningful changes, practiced over time, will create a revolution in your circumstances. This is a radical thought shift from traditional teaching.

> **Get REAL Tip:** Put to rest the idea of waiting for the "right" time to start the *big* diet, the *big* exercise routine, and the *big* "special time" for me plan.

Start by doing a little bit all the time. Avoid up-and-down patterns where one day you surpass goals and the next day you don't even meet them. Make a conscious effort to add a few healthy habits and consistently practice them—things like adding in small episodes of exercise, making a few better food choices, or doing a few minutes of quality reading for mental well-being—and become content with that.

You are supposed to enjoy life, not dread it or feel bad about not doing certain things. Begin to accept the joy moderation can bring. Decide to accept not being perfect, and you will begin to see some long-term results. Don't stay on that up-and-down roller coaster of doing well for a while when things are good, then chucking it all when it is no longer new or convenient.

Being accountable for your choices is a good place to start. Choose either a person, group, or personal chart to keep you doing what you say you want to do. Accountability creates consistency. You are more likely to keep making small changes and less likely to skip them now and then. Skipping tends to start a negative downward spiral that leads right back to where you are now. The spins, twists, and turns always lead you right back to where you started from. Are you ready to get off the roller coaster and embrace the slow and steady Turtle Power? Remember, life is a journey, and you need to enjoy the ride!

> **Get REAL Point:** Total wellness takes a combination of:
> - *Intentional* dietary choices (not just restriction)
> - *Consistent* increased activity
> - *Regular* personal development

Many people who struggle with healthy living face emotional issues that interfere with reaching their goals. The group Emotions Anonymous has a credo that could help people who face these kinds of roadblocks. By regularly affirming these truths, emotional issues can be overcome. You can use the following credo to reaffirm that each day is a choice. By tackling each day as it comes, you will no longer be overwhelmed by how hard it will be to keep up your healthy choices over the long run. That kind of thought shifting can help keep you on track.

Emotions Anonymous Credo: "Just For Today"

JUST FOR TODAY I will try to live through this day only, not tackling my whole life problem at once. I can do something at this moment that would appall me if I felt that I had to keep it up for a lifetime.

JUST FOR TODAY I will try to be happy, realizing that my happiness does not depend on what others do or say, or what happens around me. Happiness is a result of being at peace with myself.

JUST FOR TODAY I will try to adjust myself to what is—and not force everything to adjust to my own desires. I will accept my family, my friends, my business, my circumstances as they come.

JUST FOR TODAY I will take care of my physical health; I will exercise my mind; I will read something spiritual.

JUST FOR TODAY I will do somebody a good turn and not get found out—if anyone knows of it, it will not count. I shall do at least one thing

38

I don't want to do, and will perform some small act of love for my neighbor.

JUST FOR TODAY I will try to go out of my way to be kind to someone I meet; I will be agreeable; I will look as well as I can, dress becomingly, talk low, act courteously, criticize not one bit, not find fault with anything, and not try to improve or regulate anybody but myself.

JUST FOR TODAY I will have a program. I may not follow it exactly, but I will have it. I will save myself from two pests—hurry and indecision.

JUST FOR TODAY I will stop saying "If I had time." I never will "find time" for anything. If I want time I must take it.

JUST FOR TODAY I will have a quiet time of meditation wherein I shall think of God *as I understand Him* and of my neighbor. I shall relax and seek truth.

JUST FOR TODAY I shall be unafraid. Particularly, I shall be unafraid to be happy, to enjoy what is good, what is beautiful, and what is lovely in life.

JUST FOR TODAY I will accept myself and live to the best of my ability.

JUST FOR TODAY I choose to believe that I can live this one day. The choice is mine!

PART II

CREATE A HEALTHY OUTLINE

CHAPTER 4

Building Your Own Personal Wellness Plan

What drives you? What keeps you going through the day? What do you look forward to doing? These are important questions. We all live a "purpose-driven" life, whether we realize it or not. However, in looking at most lifestyles, the purpose would seem to be pleasure, self-indulgence, self-preservation, or just working toward the point where nothing "has to" be done. Step back—look at your life. What is the purpose of each thing that fills your time? What do you get from it? What is the payoff? Understanding the reasons you do the things you do is an important part of making any permanent change.

> **Get REAL Point:** When you find real purpose in an activity, you will have energy for it! You will carve out time to do it.

When it comes to healthy behavior, do you manage well while in the routine at work, but during the evenings or weekends lose focus? Often this lack of purposeful direction can cause an uneasy feeling that leads to food consumption to reduce that unpleasant sensation. Increased unhealthy food consumption can also lead to a negative energy balance, and so the downward spiral begins. It may be that you have plenty of things you could do or even need to do, but without the comfort of your routine or the deadline pushing you, you are unable to settle on the best use of your time.

Lack of a relevant purpose for your activity can lead to a form of boredom that causes emotional eating and depression. To combat this, you must find a meaning behind what you are doing to fill your time. If you fall victim to this scenario, developing a clear goal-purpose-outcome connection can result in the reduction of negative coping behaviors such as junk food consumption. So it goes with incorporating healthier behaviors. To continue the behavior in the long term, you must know your goal, have a clear purpose for doing it, and greatly desire the outcome.

> **Get REAL Note:**   You must develop a *passionate purpose* for your changes or you will not stick to them.

Begin to find your purpose and passions and live inspired. Living inspired is a state of mind that you choose. When you find your passion and create a vision, each day takes on new meaning. This allows you to wake up energized, knowing you have the opportunity to make strides toward your goals. You are eager and willing to step out and act on your convictions and ideas.

When you operate within your zone of passion, others cannot help but catch that enthusiasm. You can become a beacon of inspiration to others as you pursue your goals. We are each born with a purpose—an inspiration, a reason that makes us want to get out of bed each morning. Find yours.

Get REAL Concept 4:
Set your goals and determine what you will get from their achievement.

Goals must be realistic and achievable—short-term and long-term. You need to decide what you want to achieve through adopting a healthier lifestyle. This is very important and will determine your approach in achieving your goals. You can't hit your target if you do not know what you are aiming at or why you are aiming at it.

> **Get REAL Point:** You will make changes when you believe the payoff is worth the effort and sacrifice of changing your habits.

Write down your goals and put them where you will see them. This measure gives them solidity and increases the likelihood that they will be achieved. Determine how important it is for you to meet these goals. Your goal could be to lose a number of pounds, lower cholesterol, improve health, or just to look and feel better. Whatever it is, it must be worth enough for you to change your habits and lifestyle. If it is not, then cut yourself some slack and accept who and how you are now. Don't feel guilt and condemnation over not doing those behaviors that you think you should be doing. Remember, don't *should* on yourself! When your situation or mindset changes, then you can evaluate if the time is right for change. Until then—release guilt.

> ✔ **MY part:** provide blueprints to achieve a healthier lifestyle.
> ✔ **YOUR part:** read the information, *consider* how it applies to you, and then *commit* to doing those things you have learned.

Get REAL Concept 5:
Choose changes that are realistic and only minimally painful.

When you start with small, manageable changes, you are more likely to stick with them and build on that success. Starting small also creates an easier transition into a permanent lifestyle change. It allows you to enjoy the journey and appreciate the benefits of a healthier lifestyle.

Think of life as a marathon, not a sprint. Most people start out fast and strong, but run out of steam in the end. You are in training for your life marathon. That means starting slow and gradually increasing your tolerance.

Now is the time. Discover your purpose and choose the best path to reach your goals. Write it down, map it out, and follow it to start living a healthier life now. Current theory is so rigid and unobtainable that it saps your energy and motivation.

No wonder people try it, hate it, and ultimately fail. When you start a gung-ho plan to quickly reduce weight, the struggles will come. Frustration gradually builds, and you begin to dread the healthy choices.

Many people will change their behavior begrudgingly, just to obtain a certain goal. Then as old habits are added back in, they face a systemic revolt. The complex body of hormones, chemical signals, and psychological issues attributed to deprivation and food will mutiny.

Strict, unpleasant restriction leads to overindulgence when the restrictions are lifted! This is one reason dieters tend to eventually regain lost weight. These are REAL chemical responses in the body.

Get REAL Note: To make REAL changes, you must first face what is realistic for who you are and for your current lifestyle.

Get REAL Concept 6:
Keep a daily calendar or journal of how you spend your time.

Make it a goal to write down how you spend your time for at least one week. Use one color for planning and one for what really happened. Also note how long each activity actually took. Consider this a visual wake-up call. You will be able to see where all your time goes, making it easier to find where bad habits are hiding and where good habits can be scheduled. It reveals much about how you are really living life. By visually mapping your time, you can see what is stealing your precious energy.

Most of us do not plan time for ourselves. We take what is left over. Often that time is squeezed out, because we are not realistic about how much time other activities will take. We plan our time as we would *like* things to go, not how they most likely *will* go.

This is a big problem for most people, especially me! This is an issue I constantly battle, even though I full-well know better! I must remind myself—planning accurate time for things gives me the gift of time. It also allows me to be more peaceful and less frazzled.

Often people do not make an honest appraisal of how time is spent. You need to evaluate whether you spend your time on those things you say matter most to you. Seeing how you budget time can be an eye-opening realization and reveal areas that need to be changed in your schedule. Many people find they are "over budget" and are "spending" in the wrong areas. As always, this information is only as good as your willingness to do something about it.

> **Get REAL Note:** Having time for yourself is essential to your mental and physical health. If it is neglected, you will pay for it in stress, burnout, and dissatisfaction.

Stress is everywhere! In the "pursuit of happiness," Americans push the envelope, forgetting how to just *be*. After all, we are human beings, not human doings. Many feel the need to be doing something constantly. If they take even a small break to stop and enjoy what they have accumulated, they feel guilt. People spend so much time accumulating things that they don't have the energy or mindset to enjoy them.

When was the last time you just sat and enjoyed a peaceful moment relaxing, without having the TV on or actively doing something? Americans struggle to have it all. That is never possible. In the pursuit of many goals, something will have to be compromised to keep all of the plates spinning. This lifestyle can be brutal to your physical and mental well-being. This constant state of motion and activity leaves your system run down and ill equipped for relaxation.

> **Get REAL Point:** You create your lifestyle. Many things about your day can't be changed, but other things are choices.

Even when the purpose of a choice or activity is noble and good, if it pushes you beyond your limits, it will cause stress. This stress is literally killing people. Most doctor visits are a direct result of stress-related illness, so either plan now or pay later!

When stressed, people don't want to try new things. They want to just "get by," not change to healthier habits. After all, the unhealthy habits are used to self-soothe and comfort. Practiced over time, this negative pattern contributes to numerous health problems. These don't develop overnight. They result from years of poor choices and habits. The constant hectic and hurried pace people maintain causes metabolic imbalance and adrenal fatigue.

When a person experiences stress, the body releases cortisol and adrenalin into the bloodstream. This serves a purpose during fight-or-flight situations. The problem comes when a person remains in that state without recovery time. This causes metabolic burnout and has resulted in much of the substance abuse we see today. People need nicotine, alcohol, prescription medication, drugs, or caffeine just to keep it all going. People look for something to help them wake up, something to let them sleep, and something to keep going throughout the day.

Many conditions, such as heart disease, anxiety, fibromyalgia, chronic fatigue, depression, and elevated cholesterol or blood pressure, are affected by prolonged exposure to stressful living. This reaction to stress has even been dubbed "Hurry Sickness." Many Type A individuals hear a message like this and think "yes, that is right." They write words like "relax" and "simplify" on their already full to-do lists. That is what the concept becomes—something else to do, instead of what it was intended to be, which is a reason to change the pace and focus of one's time.

This is not an issue of simply doing things differently; it involves approaching how you live life from a different angle. It is only through a purposeful shift in thinking that chronically stressed and busy people will make smarter choices. Start by using these tools.

The Five Get REAL Steps for Stress Management

- Recognize what is too much.
- Schedule *equal* recovery time for periods of overactivity or stress-causing events.
- Say NO to having more things—YES to having more free time to just *be* and not *do*.
- Constantly assess for imbalances, and be flexible to make needed changes.
- Allow time for self-expression and creative pursuits, which create healthy energy.

So now what? Everyone is exposed to stress. The mission becomes to improve your reaction to it. Just because a stressor is encountered does not mean that you must begin stressing about it. This situation comes down to choice. You must choose daily what you will allow into your life and what you will allow to create stress in you.

If you are feeling beat up and run down, that is a signal it is time to stop and reevaluate your current choices. Continue to push, and your body will send a clear message to slow down, forcing you to take better care of yourself. It is called sickness.

Take steps now to protect yourself. Physical and mental health can be improved through awareness, planning and purposeful stress management. A little planning and sacrifice now can pay huge dividends for your future. Be mindful, live in the now, and take time regularly to just *be* in the moment. Notice the beauty around you, and allow yourself to experience simple relaxation!

Get REAL Tip:	Plan time each day to look forward to something positive. Whatever you do to de-stress, practice it regularly and look forward to it as your special time. The "look forward to it" part is key. Investing in yourself is always worth the effort. The return on that investment will pay healthy dividends in every aspect of life.

There are only so many hours in the day, and trying to add without taking something away becomes a burnout issue. It is good to visualize how you spend your time. Organizing a schedule is much like organizing a closet. There is room for only a certain number of items before it becomes too full to find anything.

So it is with your time. You need to visually see where all of your time goes. Whatever your issue is, it can be uncovered by keeping your calendar or time journal. From there, you can make small changes to chip away at problem issues.

You also need some room left to move things around. This is called *margin*. Margin needs to be built into your schedule. It is a REAL challenge to say no to back-to-back activities. Allowing a nonnegotiable buffer time between each activity will pay huge dividends when things do not go as planned. For me, getting started is always an issue. To get somewhere on time, I need to schedule a "start to get around" time and build in an extra thirty minutes in front of that.

No time for you? Then you need to prune from your schedule the activities that no longer bear fruit or reward you. If the activity does not line up with your "What Matters Most" list, or you no longer get the "fruit" from it, look for ways it can be gracefully removed. As your schedule is opened up, you can begin to schedule time for personal improvement activities that recharge the batteries, such as walking, exercising, or reading.

> **Get REAL Tip:** If an activity or duty does not bear "fruit" in your life, consider "pruning" it so YOU can grow!

Relaxation time and hobbies can help people become happier and more personally fulfilled. Freeing up time by dumping unproductive time-sappers will help you regain control of your life. You may then see the "fruit" of your better choices. But don't wait to start making better choices. Begin by doing what you can do—now. The roots you spread will affect your ability to grow.

To achieve better physical health, it is important to protect your mental health. In order to safeguard your sanity, you must create healthy boundaries. Boundaries serve two main purposes. Just like a traditional fence, they keep out what you don't want in your space, and keep safe what you do want in your space. For many different reasons, it is often difficult to set boundaries.

With the constant barrage of stimulus we encounter daily, it becomes necessary to filter the incoming information and emotions you are confronted with. Setting boundaries gives you the power to control the gate and allow into your life only what is useful and beneficial. It also gives you the authority to shut the gate on people, information, and behaviors that are harmful to you and your goals.

Creating personal boundaries is important when people make demands on your time. You need to have clear guidelines to measure against when deciding how to spend your time. By establishing your personal time boundaries up front, you will be able to make more beneficial and consistent decisions. You will have a clear-cut "yes" or "no," based on whether the activity lines up with the criteria you have set for yourself. These should be based on your "What Matters Most" list and personal values.

Today's society has become so fast-paced that people are "plugged in" 24/7. You are accessible by cell phone, e-mail, or even GPS. This constant accessibility can be a blessing and a curse. In a crisis or emergency, having a cell phone is a blessing. When you are trying to relax, getting numerous messages requesting your reply can be a curse. It is not necessary to be constantly bombarded by electronic intrusions.

Get REAL Note: Seek ways to create balance in your day so that you can be fully present in each moment.

You need to create times in your day that are technology free. This will require you to set boundaries and stick to them. This unplugged time can become a haven in your day. The first step is to notify those who regularly make demands on your time. They may not like it, but they need to realize how setting boundaries will help you organize each day and reduce your stress. Use this breakdown to help you set some healthy technology boundaries.

The Five Get REAL Steps for Technology Boundaries

- Set aside a specific time of day when calls will be returned. Don't answer your phone at home during specified family times. It's okay—really. Callers can leave a message, and you can get back to them during your specified time.

- Limit checking the computer, electronic planner, cell phone, or e-mail to once or twice a day at set times. Don't gasp! If you want to get really crazy—try scheduling some days off!

- Answer your cell phone only when expecting a call or during specified call-back times. Remember you have a choice—live in the present and tangible moment.

- When spending time with people, please don't use these technology devices. Use common courtesy and give your full attention to the person you are with. Through technology dependence, society is learning to *devalue* actual human contact. It is no wonder there has been a rise in attention deficit disorders! Technology encourages people to regularly do multiple things at once.

- If you must use a cell phone or text while in the company of others, step aside and asked to be excused. Otherwise it can be very awkward for those around you to have to listen to your conversation—not to mention that making people play second fiddle to an electronic device is rude.

By the way, take a Get REAL gut check—how uncomfortable are you feeling right now? Technology detox may be difficult for you at first. Many people have become addicted to their 24/7 technology fix. I call it "techno-excess syndrome." You may want to wean yourself gradually, or you may decide to go cold turkey into your new plan. As always, it will depend on you. The main purpose of this step is to address the subject and deal with it appropriately.

> **Get REAL Bottom Line:**   Take back control of your life, and remember to fully *live* in the moment!

PART II

SELECT A NUTRITION STRATEGY

CHAPTER 5

Eating for Life:
Creating a Concept You Can LIVE With!

You must learn to eat purposefully, and if you don't enjoy the food, don't put it in your mouth. Enjoy the calories you eat; savor them. Slow down—cut your food into small pieces and put your fork down between bites. Enjoy conversation with meals, and relax. Calories are necessary for life; they are fuel. Choose food by considering what it does for your body. When you give your body what it needs, you can then confidently add some "pleasure foods"—guilt free.

Get REAL Concept 7:
Discover the non-diet approach.

The non-diet approach includes learning about what portions really are and learning to budget foods according to your nutritional needs. This will require you to estimate portions, evaluate nutritional content, and read labels. For a while, record this information each time you eat or drink. It is a reality check about what you are actually consuming and when. After a while, you will be able to gauge, quite well, what you are taking in without thinking much about it. When you do this, no foods are "bad" or off-limits. All foods have a place in your outline.

You are in the driver's seat. You make choices according to your preferences and nutritional needs. This allows you to listen to your body's natural cues again. It will require you to educate yourself and pay attention to what you are eating, when you are eating, and what food groups you are pairing. You will also need to determine whether you are carbohydrate sensitive. This will greatly influence your food planning choices. Learning about your current habits will allow you to reshape the way you approach eating. To understand this concept better, take a look at this three-phase plan.

Three-Phase Get REAL Nutrition Plan

Nutrition Phase I has two goals: create awareness and expand your knowledge. *Keeping an intake log is absolutely the best way to do this.* By doing so, you will develop the skills needed to make informed choices. Perhaps more importantly, keeping an intake log creates accountability and a record from which to see areas for improvement.

When planning your daily consumption, it is important to determine your actual caloric needs. The larger your current body size, the greater your caloric needs will be. As you lose weight, you will have to reduce the amount of food you take in or increase the amount of energy you burn through exercise. Combining diet and exercise yields the best results over time.

Most people have no idea how many calories they consume on an average day. In order to start making smarter choices, you need to accurately see where you are now. This involves keeping track of how many calories you take in *for a short time*. Account for everything you eat and drink during the day. Be sure to note in your log what you took in, how much, and when.

Look up the approximate number of calories and note the food groups. You may use the Internet or any calorie book at the library to find out this basic information. Many restaurants also provide calorie counts on-site or on their website. This information will slowly begin to reveal how you got where you are now.

Weight Loss Formula:	To lose one pound in a week, you must burn approximately 3,500 calories over and above what you already burn doing daily activities. If you can burn an extra 500 calories per day or reduce 500 calories from your diet, you'll lose one pound a week. Focusing on small daily changes, in both diet and exercise, yields the best results. You won't lose weight overnight, but you are more likely to create permanent change.

Calorie approximation takes time to become good at. Use your best judgment and estimate until you get better at it. Err on the side of more calories when in doubt. Multi-ingredient foods are especially tough, but you are not being tested. This is only a tool to help you see how much you are taking in. It can be an eye-opening exercise!

Most people take in many more calories than they realize. By budgeting your calories throughout the day, you will have a better understanding of what a sensible meal would consist of. Intake logging allows you to see the big picture. It creates an awareness that leads to better food planning. This will help you determine ways to trim your calorie intake and change your food choices so that you can achieve REAL results.

PHASE I Nutrition Questionnaire

 Become aware of your current eating habits.

- How many calories do you consume on a regular basis?
- Do you regularly exclude certain food groups?
- Do you eat mostly processed or convenience foods?
- Do you frequently overindulge in high-calorie foods?
- Do you have emotional triggers that cause you to crave eating to soothe those feelings?
- Does being overweight create a "payoff" for you (such as allowing you to hide or be left alone)?
- Are there times of day that seem to be more difficult for you to make good choices?
- Do you balance your consumption of sugar or simple carbohydrates with a protein or complex carbohydrate?

 Learn more information about healthy eating.

- How many calories do you need to consume to maintain your current weight? How many to lose one pound per week?
- How many portions of each food group make up your healthy calorie range?
- What is an actual portion of each food group?
- What are the basic exchanges (equal calories per serving) for each food group?
- How many calories are in each basic food group serving?

- What would constitute a balanced meal choice based on your caloric and nutritional needs?
- What can you do to make better choices when balancing your food options?

Phase II Nutrition takes all the information you have learned and shapes it into a useful food plan. Starting from your current average calorie intake, begin to decrease that by 10 percent weekly. A rapid decrease is extremely difficult to maintain and often leads to overindulgence due to the unnatural over restriction. This can be self-defeating in the long run.

Your body perceives a dramatic decrease in calories as a possible famine, and this causes the release of fat-storage hormones. Gradual decrease is effective because the body is designed for this kind of self-preservation. To achieve lasting weight loss, you need to work with this survival principle.

> **Get REAL Note:** Use the same 10 percent rule when increasing your activity output. This means you will gradually make changes by only 10 percent each week.

This moderate plan allows you to ease into changes and increases the likelihood you will stick with them for the long term. First you will need to determine where you are currently. Then make your goal to decrease your calories by 10 percent this week, another 10 percent the next week, and so on until you reach your goal range.

The same goes for increasing activity. Add 10 percent more time or 10 percent more weight until you reach your goal range. Choosing a range versus a specific number gives you more flexibility and freedom to live a REAL life with some boundaries as guidelines.

When considering what calorie level will produce weight loss, a good rule of thumb is to multiply your current weight (in pounds) by ten. Be aware that as you lose weight, this number will also need to decrease. An exception to this rule would be someone who weighs 120 pounds or less. It should never be recommended to go lower than 1,200 calories without medical supervision. Knowing what is a reasonable number of calories to take in will allow you to make smarter, better planned choices.

Another consideration in the equation is your level of activity. It is important to realize the value of activity in maintaining a healthy lifestyle. The more active you are, the more calories you can consume. Activity affects calorie balance—energy in versus energy out. It is not necessary to only limit calorie intake. You can increase your activity level and see progress as a result of using more calories than you take in. This results in actual weight loss.

> **Get REAL Note:** To maintain her current weight, a woman finds she should be taking in 2,200 calories per day at her current activity level. But after keeping a food journal, she finds that she's actually taking in 2,450 calories daily. By consistently taking in 250 more calories per day than her body needs, she could gain one pound every two weeks! That would continue until her new weight ballooned to allow those calories as part of its maintenance number. If she decreases 250 calories per day, she could lose one pound in two weeks. This shows how easy it is to gain or lose weight without even knowing it. You can start losing weight now by consistently making a few simple changes.

Phase II is a time of disciplined eating. You must be aware of what you are eating, in what quantity, and with what other foods. Planning is a vital part of this. You need to plan your meals to ensure that you balance your nutritional intake. If you do not plan ahead, it is difficult to get all the needed servings of nutritious food.

Often, impulse choices and convenience foods take the place of more healthful ones. This happens due to a failure to plan. Just keeping the information in your head or doing hit-and-miss logging will not give you the results you desire. A commitment to intake logging and an accountability partner are solid steps toward reaching your goals.

There is another rule to consider when lowering calories. After seventy-two hours, your body begins to sense the chance of famine and will begin to actively store fat. At this point, you will need to increase your food intake by 200 to 400 calories per day in order to halt the secretion of fat-storage hormones.

After three to four days, you can decrease back to your goal calorie range. By following this three-day plan, you can work with your body chemistry instead of against it. You can more safely achieve your goal without deprivation or hormonal upsets.

I recommend that you develop a few sample menus for "go-to" meals based on your personal choices. Pick foods that you eat often and always have on hand. Be sure to balance the meal to meet your nutritional needs and perhaps even pair it with your other daily choices to make entire nutritionally balanced days. When you have met your goal, you are ready for Phase III.

Phase III Nutrition is maintenance. Once you reach your goal weight, you no longer need to log each meal. By this time, you have a solid grasp of healthy eating and have developed good meal planning skills. Now you will need to establish the number of calories required to maintain your current weight and stick to that range. Your weight will fluctuate, as is common in life. Holidays and special events often bring about a rise in weight.

It is recommended that you weigh weekly. When you reach five pounds above your goal weight, begin to use your Phase II skills to bring your weight back to your goal. At this time, weight should not be your focus, but you will need to monitor it to keep it from creeping back.

Chances are, if you have struggled with weight, you will always need to keep track of it. Once you stop paying attention, old habits are likely to return. Keeping your weight issue "on the radar," but not as your focus, is a part of your lifetime wellness lifestyle.

Get REAL Concept 8:
Just as you budget your time, learn to budget your nutritional intake.

Once you have familiarized yourself with the idea of budgeting your nutrition, you will see the structure and personal control it gives you. You have x number of portions per food group to work with. This is based on the calorie level you choose. How you divide those portions throughout the day is your choice. In doing this, you will ensure that you take in enough healthy foods to provide nutritional balance.

> **Get REAL Point:** When you give your body what it needs, it will work more efficiently to do what you ask it to do.

Be sure to include as many whole or natural foods as possible. These are foods that are unaltered and in their natural state: fresh fruits and vegetables, whole grains, and grass-fed meats. These "live" foods contain an abundance of nutrients that your body recognizes and can readily use.

By focusing on adding nutrition instead of subtracting unhealthy foods, you will likely achieve both. According to the universal "Law of Attraction," we tend to attract to ourselves that which we dwell on. Therefore, it makes no sense to constantly think about what we do not want to have.

Spend energy determining ways to get more nutrition into your daily routine. Once your body feels fully nourished, it can begin to release some of the fat it has been holding on to "just in case." The "just in case" is the survival mechanism that uses stored fat for nutrients when the body senses famine or undernourishment. The body will hoard fat when it is undernourished—not *underfed*, but *undernourished*.

In the non-diet approach, all foods are legal. There are no "good" or "bad" foods. While some foods provide more nutritional value, those that don't—but taste great—are still important. They address the mental aspect of eating and nutrition. They serve to reduce the feelings of deprivation that many people face when changing their eating habits.

In the non-diet approach, all foods are acceptable when eaten in moderation and in balance. Many people feel guilty about eating so-called "bad" foods. When you attach a value to food, it can cause unnecessary guilt or a false sense of accomplishment. This works against you and can keep you from getting back on or staying on track. A balanced eating approach allows for moderate indulgences.

This system gives you freedom within boundaries. It provides an outline for you to fill in the details. This way of eating will teach you healthy methods to balance the food you have available to you. No food lists, recipes, or meal plans—food you have, eat, and are regularly offered.

> **Get REAL Note:** Some people *must* change their diet or avoid certain foods due to specific health conditions. That is not what I am talking about when I say, "No food is off-limits." That situation is much more difficult to address. Certain health conditions will force your hand and make you look for creative ways to alter your diet. This must be done to maintain good health. Seeking out a dietitian to assist with meal planning is a smart idea for that situation. To help you make better food choices, some grocery stores and hospitals offer this service for free. Also, meal planning guides and online support groups can be a great place to get ideas associated with your particular medical condition.

Many people enjoy eating out but associate it with being "bad" or eating "illegal" foods. Fortunately, it is very possible to eat a regular meal in a restaurant. You don't need to forego your favorite foods or eat before you go out with friends or family. The same decision-making process occurs whether you eat at home or go out to a restaurant.

Many people think that they have two options when eating out: eating for taste and pleasure or eating for health. As you learn and practice healthy eating techniques, these two options will become one and the same. You don't want to feel restricted to the "healthy-living options" when eating out. That will leave you longing for the day when you can eat normally again. You should be able to order your favorite dish and enjoy it guilt free. How? By incorporating it into your plan.

> **Get REAL Tip:** Avoid assigning a value to food. If you identify a food as either "good" or "bad," it can create false guilt or pride over food choices.

If you're having a special "diet meal" that's different from what your family or friends are eating, you'll feel as though you're being punished. This will affect your mental health and can cause stress. Stress will release cortisol and thus affect your chemical and hormonal balance.

This example shows how intertwined mind and body really are. In order to be successful in changing your eating habits, you must look forward to and enjoy each meal you eat. This doesn't mean that you have to learn to enjoy rice cakes and celery. It means you must learn how to balance the foods you love.

Creating a balance is important when discovering a plan you can stick to for life. Healthy eating patterns can occur only when you're enjoying the foods you eat. If you're eating low-fat foods just to be healthy, but not enjoying the flavors and textures, your new food choices most likely won't be a permanent change.

However, if you begin enjoying foods and balancing meals, you're more likely to stick with it. When you learn to enjoy the process, healthy eating will become a part of your regular routine. To accomplish this you will need to develop a purposeful eating plan based on your individual needs.

Get REAL Concept 9:
Develop a purposeful eating plan.

Developing a purposeful eating plan means you will evaluate your individual nutritional needs, eating schedule, and food triggers. Based on this information, you will create clear boundaries and a tentative eating plan outline. This plan will need to be adjusted as you change body weight or as your lifestyle changes. Your plan should address your nutritional needs first. You must be aware of what the body needs to function at its best and look for ways to add those healthy foods into your regimen.

If you look at eating visually, each eating episode creates a portion of your nutritional outline. You will cross off nutritional goals as you meet them and note that in your outline. You retain the flexibility to insert or cross off items as you choose. At the end of the day, you can assess what areas may need more attention and note creative ways you met certain needs.

You may choose to track intake on paper or in your mind's eye. Written logs are much more effective, but this approach will depend on your personal commitment. Take note of simple ways you added healthy options to your routine food choices—things like eating fruit with your cereal or adding nuts, meat, or diced vegetables to your salad. These tips will be great "go-to" ideas that you may use in the future to fill in some nutritional gaps.

> **Get REAL Note:** There is no right or wrong way to eat. Healthy eating is all about motivation, balance, and flexibility.

The beauty of this method is that it is not set in stone. It is a guide. You may not meet your goals each day, but the plan is there to help steer you in the right direction. This approach should be more productive than your current method of "What am I feeling hungry for now?"

A purposeful eating plan is not meant to be rigid. It is designed to be flexible for the unpredictable events that make up REAL life. You will make choices from a more purposeful position. Before choosing what to eat, you will consider what your nutritional needs are and how many calories you want to spend at that eating episode. This will be based on your outline.

Following a purposeful eating plan will require you to be mindful of food choices. You must pay attention to what and how much you put in your mouth. Pay attention to your food combinations and not so much to whether they are the "wrong" or "right" foods.

Create a plan for eating that you can live with based on the number of calories you decide to start at. This will be determined by your 10 percent rule. When you build in the healthy options (to fulfill nutrient needs), you may then spend the remaining calories on more pleasure-based foods.

Life is not always predictable. There will be times when you eat a high-fat meal, when you eat beyond fullness, or when your schedule gets so busy that you don't work in exercise. This happens—it is normal! When it does happen, it is very important that you don't get discouraged and abandon your new, healthy lifestyle.

If you're like most people, your reaction to these diet and fitness obstacles is guilt. You feel as if all your hard work has been for nothing. "I blew it; I was doing so well. Oh well, I might as well enjoy this weekend and start over on Monday." Or even worse: "I just don't have the motivation or willpower to start over and be successful. I quit."

Feeling defeated, many people discontinue healthy living altogether and return to their old routine—until some mythical time in the future: "Maybe this spring will be a better time to start over again." This kind of scenario is diet mentality at work. Develop new thinking!

Get REAL Concept 10:
Plan for deviations.

This is REAL life, and you will stray off the path. With the non-diet approach, there is no such thing as cheating. When people feel they are cheating, they often punish themselves, causing guilt and feelings of frustration and defeat. Replacing the negative concept of cheating with the idea of "briefly straying from healthy habits" takes away the all-or-nothing emphasis on right and wrong.

Get REAL Tip:	You cannot treat every deviation from your plan as a failure.

Whatever your temptation or obstacle might be, keep in mind that moderation gives you freedom. As long as you do not have health conditions that limit food choices, embrace that freedom! If you keep moving forward and don't let guilt and discouragement stop your progress, you *will* develop improved eating and exercise habits.

Get REAL Point:	Life is full of unplanned obstacles, distractions, and temptations. Your best approach is to expect, plan, and prepare for them. Doing so will allow you to bend and not break.

Often, people choose structured programs because the structure relieves them from making choices. A properly designed program makes sense, but expecting to stick to a structured eating and exercise plan for an extended period of time without ever deviating makes no sense at all. It is actually a setup for failure. If you begin to change your habits with the assumption that any deviation from your plan will ruin it, you might as well not even begin!

Occasionally you may go over your calorie budget. You must learn that this is only a temporary deviation. At the next available opportunity, you can make a U-turn (just as a GPS navigation system would instruct you) and return to your original plan.

Your internal dialogue needs to be reset. It should calmly instruct you to make more "plan-focused" choices at the next opportunity. The GPS allows for mistakes and tries to help you correct them at the next opportunity.

You need to allow yourself to make some missteps, and then quickly correct them at the next opportunity. This will build confidence to overcome any future obstacles. When you give in to the cascading events that can follow the initial indulgence, you start a self-defeating cycle that leads you back to your comfortable and familiar ways.

> **Get REAL Note:** One day's behavior will not make or break your plan. It is a pattern of behavior that determines your outcome. Embracing this way of thinking removes guilt and condemnation from the situation.

Being mindful of your internal dialogue and inserting calm and non-judgmental direction will keep you on your desired pathway. Unfortunately, your internal dialogue is not naturally so kind. It will belittle, berate, and discourage you.

You think to yourself, "I've already screwed up my plan, so why even continue?" Recognize that this is just "stinkin' thinkin'" and reset that dialogue. Insert this new dialogue into your brain: "At the next available chance, I will make a U-turn." Keep in mind that all is not lost over one bad decision or one bad day.

No one wants to suffer through a "lose weight quick" plan only to end up heavier than before starting it. To successfully maintain weight loss, you must commit to a lifestyle that supports consistent healthy behaviors. This I know for sure. I have cycled through many patterns of hyperdiscipline and then such frustration (burnouts) that I end up choosing no personal discipline.

This all-or-nothing cycle is why many people have so little success. You can learn to live healthfully as a rule and allow yourself a few deviations from your plan. Deviation happens in the REAL world, and any plan that does not gently guide you back will send you running to the all-or-nothing land from which you came. The savvy health-conscious person realizes this and plans for it.

Get REAL Point: Ditch all-or-nothing thinking. Most people either try to work a restrictive and unpleasant plan or decide to chuck it all and make no attempt to live more healthfully. They assume that if they cannot follow their plan to the letter, they have "failed." This common way of thinking stops real progress from being made.

For the past few decades, experts have recommended a diet high in carbohydrates and low in fat. As a result, many people base the bulk of their diet on carbohydrates—starchy and sugary foods, or foods that are metabolized like sugar in the body. Some are healthy, like corn, potatoes, and whole grains, and others are not, like candies, cakes, and highly processed grains.

Since this plan has been widely embraced, we have seen the obesity epidemic increase, not decrease as experts had hoped. This type of diet often leads people to have increased cravings and leaves them feeling hungry. By pairing your foods to balance blood sugar, you can combat this common obstacle to healthy eating.

Pairing foods will require you to become a super label reader. Pay attention to the amount of carbohydrates, fiber, and protein along with the number of servings in the package. You will use this information to create your "perfect pairs."

Get REAL Concept 11:
Learn to balance meals and snacks.

Balance quick carbohydrates and sugars (the "carbage") with a protein, dietary fat, or complex carbohydrate source to sustain your blood sugar and reduce cravings. Meal balancing and meal frequency are the keys to not feeling hungry and to maintaining your energy and sanity throughout the day. The rule of thumb is what I call a "pair-to-balance" (P2B) ratio.

A serving of protein equals 7 grams, and a serving of carbohydrate equals 15 grams. This is where you start to look at food labels and note the content. For each serving of carbs (every 15 grams), you need to consume a serving of protein (7 grams). You get the picture—consume 30 grams of carbs, and you will need to pair it with 14 grams of protein to create balance.

Get REAL Tip:	Keep in mind—always eat from at least two food groups. If you must eat a cookie, pair it with a glass of milk. The protein in the milk will help to balance the carbs in the cookie.

Balance refers to the balancing of your blood sugar. Throughout the day, your blood sugar balances like a teeter-totter. Depending on the kinds of foods you eat, it can be stable or it can bob up and down, leaving you feeling like you just exited an amusement park ride. When you balance your eating, you will reduce the spikes and crashes caused by the rise and fall of your blood sugar. It is the insulin response to the carbohydrates you consumed that causes your moods to fluctuate like a roller coaster.

To avoid this common phenomenon, you need to intentionally balance the carbs-to-protein ratio. Your mind should be set on "pair-to balance"—7 grams protein to 15 grams carbs. Pay close attention to serving sizes. If you eat a sleeve of Girl Scout cookies, the amount of protein to offset that would most likely be more than you want to take in. You can see how intentional eating, using P2B, can also help keep you in check—checks and balance.

Another detail to consider is the fiber content of food. Simple carbs and sugars are usually burned up quickly for energy; that is what causes the boost and then the crash if they are not paired with protein, fat, or a complex carb. Complex carbs have greater fiber content to slow digestion and slow down the impending crash.

Fiber acts as a broom in the digestive system, sweeping out the junk as it moves through. When you look at the food label, consider the fiber content. For balancing purposes, subtract the fiber grams from the total carbs and use that number to pair your protein and create your P2B ratio.

> **Get REAL Note:** Your P2B Ratio is 7g of protein for every 15g of carbs. Aim to balance your blood sugar by keeping this ratio in mind when choosing meals and snacks.

Another consideration is *frequency*. Try to keep your carb consumption under 30 grams per two hours. This has to do with fat storage. Carbs that are not used for energy during that two-hour period are stored as fat. By limiting the amount of carbs you eat during a two-hour time period, you can reduce the amount that will get stored as fat.

This method of intentional eating can become second nature with a little practice. You do not have to get it right 100 percent of the time, but by eating more intentionally and purposefully, you can greatly reduce cravings and hunger and stabilize your moods. Using intentional eating and pair-to-balance can make living a healthier lifestyle more enjoyable. It can affect every aspect of your life.

Be sure to factor in exercise, which causes muscles to remove sugar from the bloodstream at a more rapid rate. This effect lasts for about half an hour after you stop exercising and then tapers off. Exercising can increase the number and size of the mitochondria in cells. Each body cell contains several hundred mitochondria that turn food to energy. Exercise is thought to prolong life by enlarging and activating the mitochondria, helping them clear free radicals more rapidly from the body.

Free radicals can damage cells, which can as a result shorten your life. The absence of sugar inside cells increases their ability to clear free radicals. When sugar is allowed to again enter cells, they can still clear free radicals faster because their enlarged mitochondria will be more efficient in removing them. By adding exercise to your nutritional efforts, you provide synergy to enhance overall health.

When you feel better, have energy, and your moods are stabilized, you are better prepared to live the healthier lifestyle that you have planned. Combining exercise and P2B is the method of choice for people facing insulin resistance, which is a growing problem for the "highly processed and convenience foods" generation. Before you buy your next packaged food item, turn the label over and decide how you can P2B that item. This could change your grocery list and your life forever. Give it a try!

PART VI

SELECT AN EXERCISE OPTION

CHAPTER 6

Exercise for Life: Whatever Happened to Recess?

Do you remember having recess as a child? It gave you something to look forward to. Recess gave your mind a break and allowed you to let loose some energy. You didn't think of it as having to "get some exercise." It was just fun! You played and drank in those feel-good brain chemicals—chemicals released during physical activity and from taking in fresh air and sunshine. It is time to reclaim "recess" in your current REAL life. Don't laugh! This is not about the playground, but it *is* about reclaiming some personal time. This means getting back to the basics.

> **Get REAL Idea:** Start looking for ways to "play" in your daily life. Allow time to restore and refresh your spirit!

Most people were active as kids, because activity was part of daily life. For adults, life is much more sedentary and laden with multiple responsibilities. You now have to schedule exercise like an appointment, or you tend to skip it. It is easy to allow the stressors of life to overwhelm your childhood spirit.

Adults have forgotten how to have active fun and how to just "play." The responsibilities of life start to squeeze that out of people as they age. But playing does not have to stop at a certain age. It may be reinventing things you loved at other times in your life. How does someone get back to that idea of activity being a natural part of the day, not a tacked-on task? You must plan for it.

Get REAL Concept 12:
Schedule "recess" into your day as a gift to yourself.

All you need is ten to fifteen minutes here and there to feel the benefits that "recess" provides, mentally and physically. I always secretly felt jealous of smokers. They would take their breaks regularly, go outside, and get away—a modern-day form of recess. I am *not* suggesting you become a smoker. But it is a perfect example of how to step aside and do something just for you. Most nonsmokers would stay inside and hit the vending machine, or just work through breaks. There was no activity or habit to look forward to.

Often people feel guilt when they take a break and are not actively doing something. It is time to get over it! Now is the time to accept that it is perfectly okay and healthy to just relax in the sun or quietly read a book for a few minutes. Now is the time for finding a healthy relaxation routine. *Now is the time!*

Finding healthy activities and taking small breaks will energize your day. This is essential to total wellness. It does not matter if you do puzzles, stretch, take a walk, read a book, or just sit in the sun. Fresh air and sunlight have healing properties. When possible, take time to feel the grass between your toes, listen to the wind through the trees, or see the sun reflect off the water. Finding time to be outside and appreciate nature is very beneficial.

> **Get REAL Tip:** Try a relaxation experiment. For one week, commit to a time-out in your day. Set an alarm (use your cell phone) for ten minutes. (Sit in your car if necessary.) During this time, lay back, close your eyes, and think only about your breathing. Feel your abdomen rise and fall; feel your lungs expand and expel air. Feel your toes in your shoes, and gradually consider each part of your body relaxing in its skin.
>
> You will need your alarm, because you will be sure that ten minutes has passed already. Most people feel so guilty for doing "nothing" that it is almost uncomfortable. However, if you fill that time with smoking, eating, or any other unhealthy activity, it somehow feels more acceptable. But is it really? Face your perceptions of how you spend time and allow yourself these ten minutes of downtime. After a week, I bet you will want to continue and may even look forward to it!

Whatever you choose to do as your break-time activity, allow it to refresh you. Learning what will be rewarding for you may involve a form of behavior modification and visual imagery. It is important to discover movement patterns within you that spark enjoyment. It's not as hard as you may think. Visualize children at play: some like rough-and-tumble play, like wrestling and tag; others prefer more sedentary activity, like reading or playing with dolls and action figures. What did you like?

You need to anchor fitness within the imagination. This works because feelings toward the body and its movement become entwined with self-identity. Start associating activity and movement with pleasure.

Get REAL Concept 13
Brainstorm about activities you have enjoyed in the past.

What was satisfying as a child can often be the spark to motivate you later. Using imagery, visualize your favorite games in elementary school and during middle school. Remember falling in a pile, panting heavily and laughing with friends. What were those activities?

Discover ways to reinvent them in your life today. Write down as many of those activities as you can think of. Beside them, note an activity that you could do today to recreate the feeling you gained from the behavior.

Activities I have enjoyed in the past: Ways to recreate that today:

_____   _____

_____   _____

_____   _____

_____   _____

What this mental exercise does is reawaken a positive attitude. As many people age, they get a negative attitude about exercising. They see it as a chore, something else they need to do. They stop seeing it as recess, a time to blow off steam and play. Things like the holidays and special events will come and alter their planned routine. Often they gain weight, and as a result their energy levels sink. This can cause multiple starts and stops to an otherwise healthy routine.

Most people have no desire to do tasks that they consider unpleasant, especially when undernourished and overfull. This creates an unhealthy situation—*dread.* You just don't feel like doing the activity, though you know you should. When you dread an activity, it becomes difficult to benefit from it. You need to reawaken the idea of playful activity. Here are some ideas.

If you are *run down* and you need to generate some energy, look for ways to move that involve play and not just routine exercise. Things like:

➤ Driving golf balls or practicing putting.

➤ Hitting balls at a batting cage or playing catch with a child.

➤ Calling friends for an informal pickup game of basketball, volleyball, or tennis.

➤ Playfully dancing in your living room to your favorite music, complete with air guitar and makeshift drums—that will get your heart pumping!

➤ Jumping on a trampoline or jogging on a mini-rebounder.

➤ Swaying your hips with a hula hoop or jumping rope with the kids. Try virtual exercise using a Wii.

➤ Hiking through the woods, utilizing the rough terrain. Try running up that neighborhood hill.

➤ Participating in a group exercise class, utilizing the peer pressure.

When you are *keyed up* or tense, you need de-stressing activities, not rigid exercise. You need to remove toxins and lessen your fatigue. Try things like:

➤ Stretching, yoga, or gentle rolling on an exercise ball.

➤ Slipping away to read a few chapters in a favorite book.

➤ Easy walking, meditation, or focused prayer time.

➤ Moving to music, dancing in the kitchen, or teaching kids to dance.

➤ Getting a massage, body treatment, manicure, or pedicure.

➤ Turning on soft music, dimming lights, and shutting out distractions. Utilize aromatherapy for the full effect.

➤ Lounging in a hot tub, whirlpool, or sauna.

➤ Watching a funny movie and really laughing!

When you experience apathy and feel *unmotivated*, try an activity you don't normally do to move you out of that zone. Some ideas to consider:

➤ Join a group that is active in your community or church.
➤ Exercise outdoors! Dress appropriately, breathe fresh air, and experience the extremes of nature.
➤ Take a ballroom, line dancing, square dancing, or martial arts class.
➤ Take a noncredit college class.
➤ Garden—plant some seeds or flowers. Create beauty around you.
➤ Explore a hobby or start a project that intrigues you.
➤ Learn a new game. Think like a kid—it can be fun. Allow yourself to play with the kids just for fun!

When you become *bogged down* in the same old activities, you may be ready for a change. So if you have become bored with your routine, it is time to push your body with a new challenge. Ideas to try:

➤ A high-energy exercise class, such as spinning (a group workout on exercise bikes).
➤ Interval walking (regular-paced walking combined with short bursts of an all-out sprint, followed by recovery walking).
➤ Trail hiking, not your average walk.
➤ River rafting, paddle boating, or canoeing—think paddling on the water.
➤ Cycling outdoors, inline skating, or roller skating.
➤ Walking the school track and then running the bleacher stairs.
➤ Trying a new exercise video or listening to a new audio book while walking or exercising.

Remember that activity does not have to involve an all-out effort to be beneficial. So when you consider how to spend your time, determine whether you are run down, keyed up, unmotivated, or bogged down. Choose activities based on your personal needs and your current situation.

If you are too run down—working all week, shuttling kids, and running errands—don't beat yourself up that you didn't walk or exercise that day. Instead, look forward to doing some form of activity that restores energy. This shift in thinking promotes gentle, restoration activities versus just hanging out on the couch!

On days when you have more energy, push yourself. Those are the days to try an exercise class, do interval walking, or run up and down the stadium stairs. There are many options if you look around and get out of your regular comfort zone. Be creative and make sure it's something you can have fun with.

Don't forget about parks, community centers, and the library. You can check out new videos, use audio books on your walks, or buddy up with a friend and take a class. Activity does not have to feel like an obligation. This is your life—being healthy should not seem like work. If it does, then try something different! By doing this, you can learn to feel good, mentally and physically, everyday of your life.

Being healthy is a lifelong process. It is something you must commit to for your lifetime. Knowing what to do to feel good and be healthy is not enough. Nor is starting off big and then only occasionally following your plan. The trick is being willing to do those things on a regular basis, especially when it is not convenient.

That is the struggle most REAL people have. Some people honestly do not know how to exercise or eat right. But most often, people do know—they just can't talk themselves into doing it, and herein lies the problem.

> **Get REAL Point:** Knowing something is not enough. Success comes from doing it.

Find ways to be active everyday and learn to eat healthy on most routine days. Also consider your mental and emotional health as you seek out what works for you and your situation. The ultimate challenge is to develop a lifelong way of thinking, not just quick-fix strategies.

Get REAL Concept 14:
Schedule times for "purposeful movement" into your day.

Building purposeful movement into your daily routine is a vital part of your lifetime wellness plan. Only you can decide what that purposeful movement will be. Find activities that you enjoy doing and schedule time to do it. This may be seasonal. You might walk inside during the winter and outside when the weather is warmer. Maybe you garden and do lawn work in the warm months and ride an exercise bike on cold or wet days.

Create your plan to incorporate purposeful movement into your schedule, but branch out as new opportunities arise. Some people like routine and need repetition to stay on track. Others need to change it up regularly to remain interested. You may choose a variety of exercises for your plan. The main considerations being, to think about moving all the time, choose a style that works for you, and structure your day to accommodate it.

The traditional way people look at exercise makes it become a form of drudgery. Reawaken to the fact that you can move just for the fun of it. It is important to create positive associations with movement. When you have a pleasant memory of movement, you are more likely to do it again. Use the skills you have learned in this guide to commit yourself to an active lifestyle, not just an exercise program.

> **Get REAL Note:** Using what you know about yourself to incorporate exercise into your life leads to improved long-term success.

Creating awareness about moving is essential. A pedometer is a tool that can help you monitor your daily movement. It can help detect the need to increase daily movement or provide maintenance feedback. A healthy goal is 10,000 steps per day. Start out by seeing what you log in a normal day, and then begin to purposefully add 500 to 1,000 steps per day until you reach your goal.

Research shows that you can shed sixteen to eighteen pounds a year by creating a *daily* habit of walking for half an hour in your target heart rate zone. This weight-bearing exercise also stimulates the mineral content to remain in the bone structure and thus reduces age-related bone loss, known as osteoporosis.

This kind of active movement triggers your survival response—meaning you often lose weight faster as your body feels it must lighten the load to facilitate future activity. The body was once trained to sense activity as a need to flee from danger. This caused it to release fat storage so you could flee faster and thus survive.

> **Get REAL Tip:** It is important to stop associating exercise with just calories burned. If that was the only benefit you obtained from exercise, it would seem very self-defeating.

Active movement does many things beyond burning calories. It releases endorphins that make you feel good, and it also signals your body to start working more efficiently. It turns off fat-storage hormones and signals the release of energy for you to complete needed tasks. You will also continue to burn calories at higher rate after you are done exercising. It basically unlocks the door to how your body functions.

When the body is in fat-storage mode, it tries to conserve energy. Because the body was once designed for the survival principle, it sensed long famines and would store fat for survival during that time. The body now sees a "diet" greater than seventy-two hours as a possible famine, and this triggers it to store fat and conserve energy.

Through the release of fat-storage hormones, your body is hardwired for prehistoric survival. The only problem is, we do not live in the Stone Age and we have an overabundance of food choices. The simple act of initiating active movement can be enough to signal the body to release fat. It will then give you the energy you need.

When the body feels that its very survival is based on you being able to flee from danger, it will give you what you need to do that. That means having energy and getting leaner. When you look at it that way, exercise is very worth your time.

Get REAL Concept 15:
Set a goal for your total minutes of movement for one week.

To make sure you get enough exercise, budget a certain amount of movement for the week. You can then decide how to spend that each day according to your schedule. Remember to pencil it in. Start raising your awareness and looking at where you can get at least five minutes of sustained movement (a.k.a. exercise) in so it can count toward your daily goal time.

Your goal should be at least twenty minutes per day. Look hard at the things you do daily and see what you can turn into "exercise." It does not have to be traditional exercise. It just needs to be sustained activity that elevates your heart rate—it all counts.

Get REAL Tip: Use the FIT Principle to gauge exercise benefits. These combined factors will determine what you gain from the activity.

F = Frequency of the exercise. How often do you do it?

I = Intensity of the exercise. How hard are you working?

T = Time of exercise. How long do you participate in it?

You want to aim for continuous movement done at a pace that will elevate your heart rate. In this way you can turn even regular chores like dusting and vacuuming into exercise when you consider the pace or intensity at which you do it. If you maintain the activity at a brisk pace for at least five minutes at a time, the duration will count toward your daily goal. The longer the duration with sustained intensity, the more benefit you get. Any activity that goes past twenty minutes in duration will increase the benefits.

It is important to know your goal and what you hope to get from your movement. If you are only looking for improved health, *any* exercise is better than none! Exercise should be fun, not something you equate with work. If it feels like work, you won't keep it up.

The media would have you think that losing weight or getting in shape is easy. Easy, that is, if you buy what they are selling. But the machines, gimmicks, and plans only work if you actually *use* them. Has your treadmill become just an extra closet? That's the problem—exercise requires something of you.

> **Get REAL Note:** People ask, "What is the best kind of exercise to give me the most benefit?" That is easy—it is whatever exercise you will actually make time to do regularly!

If you are looking to slim down and tone up, you will have to work harder and longer to see measurable results. The maintenance phase is not as rigid, but it still requires regular discipline. If you have never exercised or are very heavy, you can still exercise. If you can barely walk around the block, then start by doing that. Do what you can do until you are able to do more. But start today!

You can even start out by doing nothing more than playful moves, such as keeping rhythm to some great music. Snap your fingers and move your arms, legs, and hips. These simple moves will get you having fun while moving. The key is creating that association with fun and enjoyment.

How is your motivation over time? Well, I hope it is better than mine. I can't quite put my finger on what causes this, but I know that over time I have to work harder or find new activities to continually challenge me. As you will discover, you get the most benefit from an exercise you are enjoying rather than ones you dread. This has to do with the release of endorphins.

It is time to challenge your thinking and discover what keeps you interested. Using your personality and past successes as a guide, you can determine things that motivate you to continue your efforts. Try to think outside the box and discover ways to have fun with movement. When you enjoy an activity, keeping it in your schedule seems easier to manage.

Get REAL Concept 16:
Determine your internal and external motivators.

Use your internal and external motivators to enjoy your wellness activities. We move according to inborn preferences and personality. Because of this, the best exercise combines consistency with something you love to do. Get in touch with your own personal fitness instinct.

Get REAL Tip: Begin to discover what your personality type is, and then find activities to complement it.

Let this new way of thinking allow you to have a better relationship with your body. Transfer authority back to yourself when it comes to moving your body. Don't let others dictate to you based on what works for them. Personal motivators are unique to each person.

- ✓ If you are an *outdoor person*, then look for things that get you outside. Create outdoor movement opportunities.
- ✓ If you are *"other-directed"* and find yourself taking care of everyone, a buddy might keep you on task when it comes to personal fitness time. Exercise for this personality type should be social.
- ✓ If you are consistent and *routine oriented*, then a treadmill or written plan might be the thing for you.
- ✓ If you are *competitive* or motivated to win a prize, look for some competition in your area. You can sign up for a contest or race, make a simple wager with a friend, or train for a marathon. Allow the activity to draw from your competitive nature. Keeping score is a must!
- ✓ If you are *sports oriented*, try joining a league or starting a weekly pickup game. Heading out to the field, court, or other game spot is another way to practice your skills and burn some calories.

✓ If you *become bored easily* with routine, look at your "enjoyed activity" list. Pull ideas from what gives you pleasure. Mix up your activities and do whatever type you are in the mood for.

Keep in mind that the activities you choose can be seasonal—either seasonal as in weather or seasonal as in phases of life. Perhaps you take a fitness class in the winter, and then when spring comes you start walking outdoors. In the summer you may start swimming, and then you walk again in the fall. That is great! Don't limit yourself to a rigid, inflexible schedule.

Likewise, as the phases of life change, you may need to change the activities you choose and when you do them. With little kids at home, you may choose walking on a treadmill before their day begins. When they get older, you may need to work your activity around multiple busy schedules. If your job changes, that may require another alteration in the type of activity and the time you schedule it.

Remember that your life is fluid, and you need to create a plan that will readily adapt to your lifestyle at the time. It is this ability to constantly incorporate activity into your life that will keep you healthy and well. You must make activity a *nonnegotiable* part of your schedule, even when your schedule is unstable.

Get REAL Bottom Line: To achieve results, you must act on the knowledge and resources you have.

CHAPTER 7

Get REAL Resistance Training

You can easily see that resistance training is a valuable part of improving health and wellness. The multifaceted benefits will impact all areas of life. So why is it that so few choose to make it a regular part of their life?

Learning how to incorporate this type of training into your daily life is the real key. Your challenge is to learn how to do the exercises correctly and then find a way to build them into your lifestyle. A plan will do you no good if you will not realistically stick to doing it.

> **Get REAL Note:** Lasting change usually begins with a sharp break in your normal routine.

It is time to bust out of your rut. Often you must enact the change. Inserting a fitness class, personal trainer visit, weight loss group or challenge, or even just an exercise date with a friend into your schedule can jump-start your efforts and provide a new, healthy template. Just deciding to add some resistance training to your normal routine is usually very difficult to maintain for any length of time. It is also a *big* guilt producer.

Often it takes stepping out of the box to create a "new normal." A planned exercise time can also take pressure off you while you are trying to relax at home. Who has not sat on the couch thinking to themselves, "Boy—I really should get up and exercise a little"?

When you set aside a specific time for activity and stick to it, you will no longer feel pressure or guilt when you are at home, because you will have completed your obligation to the commitment. As a result, your time at home is more peaceful—you can rest, relax and restore without that nagging voice reminding you of what you should be doing. Consider it a gift to yourself. This can reduce stress, increase relaxation, and promote mental well-being all in one simple effort.

So create a breakout plan and stick to it. Even if it is a very small gesture, it will be more than you were doing before. As always, start small and add more as you feel more comfortable and confident in your efforts (keeping in mind the 10 percent rule). By gradually adding exercise to your routine, you allow it to become a regular behavior. Down the road you will be glad you did.

Get REAL Concept 17:
Determine what you hope to achieve through resistance training.

Again, this is a "know your goal" issue. Identifying what you hope to achieve allows you to better motivate yourself and set more realistic goals. So when you start to exercise, know what you want to get out of it.

If you are exercising for health benefits only, go for it; any time you spend will be helpful. Weight-bearing exercise or resistance training strengthens bones and reduces osteoporosis. This fact alone makes it a vital part of every lifestyle. In fact, it has multiple beneficial effects!

If your goal is to increase strength, realize that exercise in itself does not make you stronger. If it did, avid runners would have the strongest muscles. The actual stimulus that makes muscles larger and stronger is to stretch them while they contract. When you lift a heavy weight, your muscles stretch before the weight starts to move. The more stretch, the more damage to the muscle fibers.

It is when the muscle fibers heal after a few days that the gain in strength occurs. You become stronger by lifting heavier weights, not by exercising more. If you do too much work (too many reps), you will not be able to lift the heavier weights that make you stronger. When it comes to gaining strength, less may be more.

> **Get REAL Point:** To become strong, you need to exercise your muscles against resistance to the point of fatigue.

The only stimulus that makes muscles larger is to stretch the muscle fibers while the muscle shortens. To help you understand how muscles shorten, think of two sticks lying end to end. Then slide the sticks along each other so that they end up beside each other. Your muscle fibers work like this. When lifting a heavy weight, muscle fibers are stretched as the fiber filaments slide along each other.

The first time you lift a heavy weight, you use a small percentage of your muscle fibers—less than 5 percent. As you continue to lift and lower a weight, you bring in more fibers, until thirty to fifty seconds have elapsed. At this point, the lactic acid starts to accumulate in the muscle, reducing the number of contracting fibers. You use the most muscle fibers when you exercise them against heavy resistance for thirty to fifty seconds. That is the time that it takes to lift and lower a heavy weight slowly eight to twelve times.

This stimulus of exercising against heavy resistance is so strong that you can enlarge a muscle even while you are losing weight and other muscles are getting smaller. Pick the heaviest weight that you can lift and lower slowly ten times in a row. Stop lifting if there is pain or you cannot keep proper form. Studies show that most people will become as strong by lifting weights in one set of ten as they would by performing three sets of ten for the same weight.

> **Get REAL Tip:** If you are not sure about your form or your routine, you have some options. Seek a professional trainer for valuable feedback on your form or to build a routine for you. You can also take a class or learn with a friend. Whatever you choose, ensure you're doing the exercises properly, or you can do more harm than good!

Get REAL Concept 18:
Learn the proper way to train your muscles in order to meet your goals.

Some exercises will require heavier weights and some lighter. It depends on your ability to keep proper form. This list will provide a way to gauge the amount of weight you should use.

The Five Get REAL Tips for Choosing Weights

- If you find that after eight reps you are not challenged, you may want to go a little heavier.
- Reduce the weight used if you can't keep good form. For instance, you may use five pounds for shoulder raises, eight pounds for exercises that focus on the back muscles, and twelve pounds for biceps. Find where *you* need to be to remain challenged. (You may start with no weights.)
- Avoid using very heavy weights in the beginning, or you might have to quit due to soreness, strain, or possibly injury.
- Gradually increase the weight in the weeks to come as muscles become more conditioned. You will need to add some weight for muscles to remain challenged and to create the overload principle.
- Continue to increase weight as needed for continued definition.

Weight training to improve endurance would include high reps at a low resistance. This would be appropriate for runners or those not wanting to add any bulk or size. It will strengthen and improve the function of local muscles that will accommodate the repetitive actions of a speed sport such as running.

If your goal is increased muscle definition or a slight increase in mass, use moderate repetitions (two sets of eight or ten reps) at a moderate weight (50 percent to 60 percent of your repetition maximum). Repetition maximum (RM) is the maximal load that a muscle group can lift over a given number of repetitions before fatiguing.

Working the muscle to fatigue is important when the goal is development of definition or mass. To sculpt muscle and build mass, you would use low repetitions (one set of five to ten reps) at a heavier weight (80 percent of your repetition maximum). Those wishing to develop a lean, muscular body will need to add cardiovascular exercise to burn extra calories and utilize the existing fat stores. This will enhance the muscular look of the body.

> **Get REAL Note:** The three main keys to developing a lifetime habit of exercise are slow progression, consistency, and regularity.

To determine a starting weight, you need to find the maximum amount of weight you can safely lift, in good form, for ten repetitions. This will give you a good resistance range permitting you to progress to higher strength levels. After establishing your starting resistance, your next step is gradual progression.

Start with ten reps, and you can progress to two sets of ten. When that is no longer challenging your muscle, increase the weight and go back to one set of ten. Continue this process as you grow stronger and need more challenge to maintain and develop your strength and definition.

There is an average five pound per decade muscle loss. This means that an average sixty-five-year-old has about twenty pounds less muscle than at age twenty-five. This results in a decrease in physical capacity and metabolism. Since a pound of muscle burns over thirty calories a day, that twenty-pound decrease in muscle mass leads to about 600 fewer calories used on a daily basis. This lower energy requirement accounts for why many people put on weight with age. Although their habits have not changed, their ability to burn calories has.

> **Get REAL Point:** Without a change in exercise and diet, the average sixty-five-year-old will have twenty pounds more fat and twenty pounds less muscle than at age twenty-five, even if weight remains the same.

A sensible strength training program can make a huge difference in this problem. The stimulus for the development of strength is to create progressive resistance. The focus should be on intensity rather than duration. A goal would be to use enough resistance to fatigue the muscle you are working in fifty to seventy seconds.

In general, slow lifting and lowering movements are most effective. They are safer, create less stress on the joints, and involve less momentum. Make your aim to take two seconds to lift the weight and about four to lower it.

Get REAL Concept 19:
Commit to a resistance training schedule that
will fit your lifestyle and help you meet your goals.

If you make a commitment to weight training in order to sculpt and shape the body, you will need to gradually increase the weight used to see the inches come off and to have your jeans fit better. The lady who casually lifts two to five-pound weights on an infrequent basis does improve her health status but does little to sculpt and shape the body.

To have measurable results, you must have a regular program that works all of the muscle groups to fatigue at least twice a week. This will prevent deconditioning of the muscles. If they decondition before you lift again, you will not be able to reap the maximum benefit from your training. You build on the foundation you create through regular episodes of resistance training. Muscle that is out of shape is deficient in two things: mitochondria and contractile proteins.

Mitochondria are the tiny powerhouses that generate energy for your workouts, and the contractile proteins give the muscle its strength. Walking for just thirty minutes per day, or ten minutes three times a day, can replenish mitochondria and contractile proteins in a month. This will allow your body to function optimally, and you will generate more results for your efforts.

Always balance your training program with adequate nutrition. Be sure to maintain a nutrition and activity plan that creates a safe calorie deficit and includes some type of multivitamin and mineral supplement. A weight loss of any amount will lead to a reduced energy requirement. As a result, it will take fewer calories to meet your needs.

That is why a resistance training program is so important. It will increase your lean muscle mass and compensate for the reduced calorie needs. This increase in muscle will fuel your metabolism and allow you to eat a healthy amount of food even when you have reduced your size. With calorie restriction alone, your chances of having to eat less and less over time are increased.

Most people never fully commit to a program of progressive weight training, and as a result they fail to reap the multiple benefits. If you are wondering why your "spot" workouts are not working to tone and shape the muscles, my best guess would be one or more of these five reasons.

The Five Get REAL Reasons for Failure to See Results

- **The workouts are spaced too far apart.** Deconditioning occurs between workouts (often as soon as in seventy-two hours) and you are not able to progress in your workouts.

- **You are not lifting heavy enough weights for the muscles to "firm up."** The stress from overloading the muscles causes micro-tears inside them, and it is during their repair that the muscles become firm and shapely. Numerous repetitions at very little weight will work the muscles but will do little to firm them.

- **You start out lifting weights that are too heavy.** This leads to soreness and discouragement.

- **Your form is incorrect and not creating the desired effect.** Misalignment during exercise can cause injury along with a lack of progress.

- **You have too much fat tissue covering the muscle to see the benefit of your work.** This is especially true of the abs and arms. When you burn off the fat, you will see the muscle tone developed underneath.

Don't be discouraged. A weight training program done right will change the way you look at your body. The before and after pictures you see for diet pills show people who have done weight training! That is how they got those sculpted and tight muscles. They did not come from weight loss alone.

You don't get sculpted abs or firm legs because you lost weight with a pill. But that is what these companies lead you to believe. The pill could have helped the models shed some fat, a change which would allow you to see those hidden muscles. But to have the kind of definition seen in those ads, you *must* use resistance training!

Look close at those ads and you will see what I mean—not to mention that the "after" photos include a better-fitting swimsuit, better posture, a tan, makeup, and better lighting. So don't be sucked in by those claims. Those kinds of results happen because of work, not just magic fat-loss pills. I just thought you should know the truth about those ads. When you hear or see them, simply ignore them!

> **Get REAL Note:** Weight loss ads are staged to show an impressive result.

Don't allow yourself to be sucked into deceptive thinking. The media bombards us constantly with these ads, and they can seem overwhelming and depressing. Use the information you have learned from this guide to empower your decisions.

If you feel you need medication or other weight-loss aids, you should see a physician for a medically monitored plan and safe alternatives. Avoid over-the-counter hype! If these medications were that good, then why wouldn't everyone use them? Monitoring and follow-up are essential when using any type of weight-loss aids.

Get REAL Concept 20:
Plan to avoid adaptation by varying your workout plan.

Bodies can become accustomed to an exercise routine. This is one reason people experience a plateau or rut. Changing your routine about every six weeks will help prevent this. When you start a new exercise regime, your body responds because it is required to make numerous changes to adjust to different workloads. Your muscles are rebuilding themselves, and this consumes a large number of calories.

At some point, your body will stop adapting to the new workload; as a result, you burn fewer calories for the same activities. The more you do something, the better you get at it. As your body becomes better at performing your exercises, it will use fewer calories during the exercise.

As you get into better shape, your body is more efficient and takes fewer calories to operate. Improved health means your body has a lower resting metabolic rate and burns fewer calories during normal daily activities. Part of the reason is that your cardiopulmonary (heart and lungs) system is more efficient now and you have a lower resting heart rate. Don't let your body get used to the same exercise.

Maintain your body's adaptation period by changing the intensity, duration, frequency, and/or mode of exercise, and include interval training if necessary. This could be a good time to schedule a session with a professional trainer to move you forward in your progress. Plateaus are common when you are creating change in your lifestyle. Understanding why this happens will enable you to make simple changes to keep you seeing results down the road.

Get REAL Bottom Line:	You must change your plan as your body changes. Keeping your body challenged and engaged will help you avoid the adaptation phase.

PART V

DEVELOP YOUR LIFETIME WELLNESS LIFESTYLE

CHAPTER 8

Physical Conditioning

Both cardiovascular and resistance training are forms of physical conditioning. This is a key component of lifetime wellness. It refers to an intentional program of building strength, endurance, and stamina. Conditioning allows your body to work as it was designed to and at its optimum level.

It is important to understand how the body works and what benefit you can receive from a proper conditioning program. The concept of conditioning seems lost on most Americans. In this instant gratification society, the act of daily self-discipline for positive outcomes you may not see right away is a tough sell for many people.

> **Get REAL Note:** By learning more about what makes the body work, you can begin to fully grasp the importance of gradual and regular conditioning.

Exercise affects your heart and lungs. The heart is a muscle, but not the lungs. The lungs depend upon the movement of the diaphragm for the amount of air they can take in. The body needs oxygen for many functions, including providing energy by burning the food we eat for fuel.

Air is inhaled into the lungs, where the oxygen is removed. The oxygen is then forced into small, balloon-like red blood cells. From there the red blood cells are sent through the bloodstream to the heart, where they are pumped throughout the entire system. Good oxygen exchange is essential to well-being. The muscles, nerves, and other tissues are directly affected by it.

One objective of exercise is to strengthen muscles and improve tone. The main objective of any conditioning program is to increase the capacity of the lungs and heart (the cardiopulmonary system). Strengthening the heart and lungs allows oxygen to be fed more freely and easily through the cardiopulmonary system. This in itself will improve the muscular network so that physical acts can be performed more freely and with ease. Even involuntary systems such as the digestive system will function more efficiently.

The ratio of oxygen to food consumption is important. If they are not in proper proportion, weight and energy levels will be affected. Not enough food, and you will become too thin. Too much food, and you will become overfat. Not enough fuel, you are weak; too much fuel, you are lethargic. It is easy to see how balancing food consumption can greatly affect how you look and feel.

Some types of foods are burned up more easily than others. Any excess food fat can linger in the bloodstream and impair its flow. That dangerous fat, known as cholesterol, can stick to the interior walls of the arteries and narrow them. When this happens, blood flow is reduced, or even stopped if the artery becomes blocked.

This leads to what is called arteriosclerosis, or hardening of the arteries. The heart and brain must have oxygen to perform properly. Any impairment of blood flow that denies the heart or brain oxygen can cause a heart attack or stroke.

> **Get REAL Point:** Improving your cardiopulmonary fitness allows the body to function more efficiently and reduces your risk of age-related disease—the dreaded "My 'parts' are wearing out!" syndrome.

Regular physical conditioning can increase the capacity of the heart, lungs, and the entire vascular system. Another reason to exercise—just for the health of it! Greater capacity allows more blood to be carried throughout the body to the tissues and muscles. With greater blood flow, more oxygen can be utilized by the body. A well-conditioned person reduces heart rate and blood pressure as a result of the heart not having to work so hard.

Testing your *resting heart rate* and *recovery heart rate* are two ways to monitor your cardiopulmonary fitness and to see the REAL benefits of your efforts. Studies show that the maximum oxygen intake of moderately active men decreases from the age of twenty, by almost 8 percent in ten years. Subsequently it decreases 16 percent by age forty, 26 percent by age fifty, and 35 percent by age sixty. This natural decline of oxygen intake makes actively improving cardiopulmonary function even more important as you get older.

All muscles can be made more limber, larger, and stronger. The heart is a muscle and can be conditioned to do more work with less effort. This saves thousands of heartbeats each year and in theory would add more years to your life. Your heart can wear out from being overworked. It has been said, "People do not die so much as they gradually kill themselves."

Age comes not only from years but from neglect. Perhaps bodies do not "wear out" from overwork as much as they "rust out" from inactivity. Years of inactivity will do more damage to your body than the years themselves.

It is true that certain capabilities decline with age, but they can be greatly affected by regular conditioning. There are many fit older people and many unfit younger ones. You do not slow down suddenly in one day. Most people gradually slow down each day upon day of their adult life. You have the choice to start speeding up again and getting more out of the life you have left.

> **Get REAL Point:** Fitness is a state of being, not a matter of age. The determining factor is not how many years you have lived, but how you have lived during your years. This is what will have a greater influence on your level of fitness and general wellness.

It is important to keep your body strong and flexible. Working your muscles through activity will stretch and strengthen them. The more limber you are and the stronger your muscles, the better able you will be to perform the activities you want to do.

Fitness will even improve your posture. Physical fitness is the ability of the body to perform as close to its peak potential as possible. Your health allows you to resist or overcome injury, infection, and disease.

The lack of excess weight and the presence of flexibility, agility, strength, speed, and endurance will help you perform your daily tasks. A regular lifestyle of active movement promotes lifetime wellness. Activities like calisthenics, performed regularly, are useful because they loosen up the muscles and enable you to function more freely. This helps you avoid injury and strengthens muscles along with building endurance. Strength creates motion, but flexibility permits it. Balancing the two is part of your conditioning plan.

We don't easily change our nature in life. So it makes sense that your fitness type should match your basic nature. It is also important to understanding your approach to exercise. For years, people have been told to walk long and steady, aiming for thirty to forty-five minutes at a target heart range. However, there is REAL benefit from doing short (less than one minute) bursts of intense exercise, recovering, and then repeating that pattern (interval walking). In fact, this cyclic form of exercise can have tremendous health benefits.

A cyclic approach involves giving an all-out effort over a short period of time—like a minute. This short burst hits the fat stores more intensely. It floods the body with antioxidants and anti-inflammatory benefit during the recovery phase. Inflammation has been known to cause multiple problems in the body. Now, more than ever, we need anti-inflammatory types of exercise.

We now realize that exercise is good medicine. The changes that occur in the body during exertion and rest are restorative. History shows that our ancestors ran from predators, chased their prey, and then rested. Our physiology evolved according to these bursts of exertion and complete recovery. A cascade of healing occurs during the recovery phase.

Get REAL Point: Exertion and recovery are vital parts of any wellness plan. Building these contrasts into your schedule is essential to your long-term vitality.

Understanding this exertion and recovery approach is important. Too often we focus on the exertion side of the equation and neglect the recovery side. People tend to look at the body as a mechanical object. But the exertion and recovery approach looks at the body differently. Our endocrine, muscular, and circulatory systems are all cyclic in nature, and this type of exercise enhances the body's circadian rhythm.

If you ask someone, "Can you go hard for one minute, then rest?" most people are willing to try it. If, on the other hand, you say, "Go hard for forty-five minutes," there is a less than enthusiastic response. This short exertion followed by recovery approach, challenges our physiology and puts the highs and lows back into chemical and circulatory responses. It also can deter adaptation.

Another aspect of the exertion and recovery approach is creating sharp contrasts. Contrasts help to build healthy rhythms in our bodies. Cycles such as complete darkness followed by complete light, or being hot followed by being cold, assist the body's cyclic nature.

The prehistoric hunter-gatherer experienced these extremes each day. Today our artificial temperature control and lighting put restrictions on this natural physiology. To achieve better health benefits, we need to equally alternate these highs and lows.

All approaches to exercise can be used as tools to improve how the body functions. The changes exercise can produce on a chemical and physical level are powerful. Exercise can also help improve general feelings of well-being, promote relaxation, and improve depression symptoms.

Get REAL Note: Exercise is one of the best methods for relieving stress in the body, and stress-related illness is a huge issue.

It has been cited as a contributing factor for numerous doctor visits annually. You can use your physical activity to improve your mental and emotional health. Consider these benefits when you are looking for reasons to get out and get moving.

Exercise affects *heart rate variability* (HRV), which is the measure of time between heartbeats. It should fluctuate with every respiration. A loss of heart rate variability has been identified as a risk factor common to all causes of death. When you are young and the heart muscle is flexible, there is variance in beat-to-beat measure. As you age, chronic disorders set in, and you lose your HRV.

What these short bursts of all-out effort do is help restore that variability. It can be like "yoga for the heart" and acts as a homeopathic dose of exercise. These bursts are not enough to trigger respiratory fatigue, but are sufficient to generate the anti-inflammatory responses during the recovery phases. Be sure to take typical precautions based on your current health and fitness level. Attempt these methods only if you are medically able.

> **Get REAL Tip:** Utilize interval walking to see increased results.

For interval walking, check your pulse and take note of it. Add a short ten- to thirty-second "sprint," followed by slower recovery walking. ("Sprint" is a relative term based on your fitness level—consider your best attempt to flee if the house were on fire!) Then gradually build back to your brisk walk. Take your pulse again. When your heart rate has recovered to pre-sprint levels, you may sprint again. You will benefit from the elevated heart rate even when returning to the slower pace. Follow this pattern regularly, and you will get more benefit for your time of purposeful movement!

> **Get REAL Point:** The best time to begin a conditioning program is anytime you are willing to start seriously.

Creating an exercise incorporation plan based on the principles of physical conditioning is important. All three components—stretching and flexibility, resistance training, and cardiovascular exercise—need to work in harmony to create a healthy, balanced lifestyle.

You have seen how the body uses regular activity to improve body functioning. Now you must determine whether you are ready to develop your program for lifetime physical conditioning.

The Five Get REAL Goals of Physical Conditioning

- Maintain and improve flexibility
- Gradually build muscle tone and strength
- Build stamina and endurance
- Improve cardiopulmonary function
- Reverse or halt age-related physical deterioration

When it comes to conditioning, be steady but don't overdo it. You need to train—not strain. Strive for flexibility, strength, and endurance. Play to have fun and do your best. Try to stay competitive, but be willing to accept your limitations. Stay active to improve your mind, body, and spirit. In the short and long term, you will see improved health and happiness. Realize that the race is not always won by the swift. Often dedication and determination have their own rewards.

It does not matter what type of conditioning you do—more important is your mental approach. Learning to love the process instead of the goal alone will make life more enjoyable and rewarding each and every day. More endorphins are released when you are in a positive frame of mind. Endorphins are the body's opiates or pleasure-enhancing substances, found in the pituitary gland.

Optimum endorphin release occurs when there is harmony of mind and body. You would have a higher endorphin release when performing a simple task you enjoy than when performing a healthy behavior that you dislike but feel you need to do anyway. What is your mental approach to physical activity? Choose behaviors wisely—your attitude will affect the outcome.

CHAPTER 9

Practicing Prevention and Wellness

For optimal lifetime wellness, you need to know your current health numbers. Knowing what to watch for and learning about how the body functions will allow you to make more informed choices. For instance, *cholesterol* is a term that you hear often. What exactly is it? Cholesterol is a waxy substance your body uses to protect nerves, make cell tissues, and produce certain hormones. All the cholesterol your body needs is made by your liver. Cholesterol in the food you eat (such as eggs, meats, and dairy products) is extra, and too much cholesterol can have negative impacts on your health.

While some cholesterol is needed for good health, too much cholesterol in your blood can raise your risk of having a heart attack or stroke. The extra cholesterol in your blood may be stored in your arteries (blood vessels that carry blood from your heart to the rest of your body). Buildup of cholesterol (called plaque) in your arteries will cause your arteries to narrow and harden (called atherosclerosis).

Large deposits of cholesterol can completely block an artery. If an artery that supplies blood to the muscles in your heart becomes blocked, a heart attack can occur. If an artery that supplies blood to your brain becomes blocked, a stroke can occur. Cholesterol travels through the blood in different types of packages, called lipoproteins.

- **Low-density lipoproteins (LDL)** deliver cholesterol to the body. This is the bad stuff; you want your LDL number to be *low*.
- **High-density lipoproteins (HDL)** remove cholesterol from the bloodstream. This is the good stuff; you want your HDL number to be *high*.

This explains why too much LDL cholesterol is bad for the body, and why a high level of HDL is good. It's the balance between the types of cholesterol that tells you what your cholesterol level means.

Another part of routine cholesterol blood testing is your triglycerides. They are a type of fat found in your blood and are a major source of energy, as well as the most common type of fat in your body. When you eat, your body uses the calories it needs for quick energy. Any extra calories are turned into triglycerides and stored in fat cells to be used later.

The excess calories are stored as fat regardless of what kind of food you eat—fat, carbohydrate, or protein. If you regularly eat more calories than you burn, you may have high triglycerides. Below are the numbers you need to know!

Total Cholesterol Levels

- Less than 200 is best
- 200 to 239 is borderline high
- 240 or more indicates increased risk for heart disease

LDL Cholesterol Levels

- Below 100 is ideal
- 100 to 129 is near optimal

- 130 to 159 is borderline high
- 160 or more indicates increased risk for heart disease

HDL Cholesterol Levels

- Less than 40 indicates higher risk for heart disease
- 60 or higher reduces your risk of heart disease

Triglyceride Levels

- Normal triglyceride levels are under 150
- High levels are 200 or above

Blood Pressure Readings

- 110/70 or below is ideal
- 130/80 or above is borderline high blood pressure (hypertension)
- 140/90 or above is hypertension (increases risks for heart attack or stroke)

Now that you are familiar with what these terms mean and what they do, it is time to find out what your numbers are. This information is vital to your overall wellness and can be an indicator of your risk factors for heart disease and stroke. There are several factors that contribute to high cholesterol—some are controllable, while others are not.

Uncontrollable risk factors include:

- **Gender**—After menopause, a woman's LDL cholesterol level ("bad" cholesterol) goes up, as does her risk for heart disease.

- **Age**—Your risk increases as you get older. Men age forty-five years or older and women age fifty-five years or older are at increased risk of high cholesterol.
- **Family history**—Your risk increases if a father or brother was affected by early heart disease (before age fifty-five) or a mother or sister was affected by early heart disease (before age sixty-five).

Controllable risk factors include:

- **Diet**—The saturated fat and cholesterol in the food you eat raise total and LDL cholesterol levels.
- **Weight**—Being overweight can make your LDL cholesterol levels go up and your HDL levels go down.
- **Physical activity/exercise**—Increased physical activity helps to lower LDL cholesterol and raise HDL cholesterol levels. It also helps you lose weight and maintain healthy blood pressure.

Knowing your numbers and monitoring them regularly should be a major part of your lifetime wellness lifestyle. This and regular blood pressure readings, an annual physical, and age-appropriate screenings are vital to overall health and wellness. If you have known risk factors, then it becomes even more important for you to stay on top of your health and keep a check on your health status. When you know what you are working with, you can take active measures to ensure your best health now.

Get REAL Point: The old adage is true—"An ounce of prevention is worth a pound of cure."

Here are "25 for 5": twenty-five ideas to create the five following life-time wellness lifestyle changes:

- ✓ Improve total cholesterol
- ✓ Lower LDL cholesterol
- ✓ Raise HDL cholesterol
- ✓ Lower triglycerides
- ✓ Reduce blood pressure

1. **Make lifestyle changes to reduce stress.** Learn better ways to cope with the stress you encounter. Stress management is essential to regulate delicate chemicals and hormones in the body.

2. **Lose weight or maintain it close to your ideal weight.** Staying at a healthy weight allows your body to work more efficiently and reduces many negative risk factors.

3. **Be physically active daily.** Aim for at least twenty to thirty minutes of physical activity a day, or fifteen miles of walking per week.

4. **Stop smoking, or don't start!** Avoid secondhand smoke when possible.

5. **Enjoy whatever activity you choose.** Studies show that the mind-body connection is powerful and affects your total health, either for better or for worse.

6. **Eat more soluble fiber.** Achieve this with fruits, vegetables, whole grains, and beans—especially oats, barley, and prunes. Soluble fiber actually removes cholesterol from your bloodstream.

7. **Add oat bran to your diet.** It has a unique ability to naturally lower cholesterol. There is something to be said for those Cheerios!

8. **Eat intentionally.** Eat so that you take in the nutrients that your body needs to function optimally. Don't exclude the foods you love that don't meet that description—just limit how often and how much you indulge in them.

9. **Get plenty of fluids.** Not just water—drink juice, low-fat milk, and other beverages liberally throughout the day.

10. **Try psyllium** (such as Metamucil). Use it as a supplement, ideally one teaspoon in a large glass of water before each meal.

11. **Eat more whole grain.** Aim to reduce your servings of refined "white" grain products.

12. **Take a daily aspirin.** An 81-milligram baby aspirin is sufficient, with a twice monthly booster of 325 milligrams. Bedtime is the optimum time to take aspirin. Ibuprofen (such as Advil or Motrin) may block the effectiveness of aspirin. An alternative for pain relief is naproxen (Aleve or Naprosyn)—it adds to aspirin's ability to prevent clotting.

13. **Cook with real garlic.** Avoid the garlic supplements, which have not been shown to work. Real garlic acts as a natural blood thinner.

14. **Try phytosterols** (plant sterols). They have been shown to block the absorption of cholesterol. Supplements are hard to find, but butter replacements such as Benecol and Take Control will give you an additional LDL reduction when used regularly.

15. **Eat fruits and vegetables from a wide variety of sources and colors.** Each food and color offers different health benefits. Changing it up and eating a variety are keys to healthy nutrition.

16. **Try a glass of red wine or beer.** Studies show that for adults, *moderate* daily consumption can have significant health benefits. ("Moderate" means two drinks per day for men, one for women.) More than that amount will not increase the benefits and can lead to other health problems. *Note:* This would not be recommended for everyone.

17. **Cut back on saturated fats and trans fats.** Avoid trans fats whenever possible.

18. **Embrace healthy fats.** The fat in foods such as nuts, olives, avocados, fatty fish, and olive oil will improve your HDL and can help reduce total cholesterol. Make an effort to add these to your diet, but use moderation on portions. It is easy to overdo it.

19. **Try to eat fish at least twice a week.** Fish is rich in valuable omega-3 fatty acids.

20. **Start taking niacin.** Niacin, also known as vitamin B_3, helps stop the body's excess production of cholesterol in the blood. It also raises HDL and lowers triglyceride levels. Supplementation is recommended in a gradual method, not to exceed 3,000 milligrams (if you use the immediate release form) or 1,500 milligrams (sustained release) daily. Not increasing gradually can lead to flushing. It is best to take the niacin at mealtime with food and plenty of fluids. Taking your aspirin prior to the niacin eliminates or weakens the flushing. Niacin has been noted to have a major influence on lowering cholesterol.

21. **Try the supplement pantethine.** It is a derivative of panothenic acid and can dramatically raise HDL and lower triglyceride levels.

22. **Take B vitamins daily.** They control the buildup of the amino acid homocysteine. You can take a B complex or individual vitamins: B_6, 2 milligrams; B_{12}, 6 micrograms; and folic acid, 400 to 800 micrograms.

23. **Supplement with omega-3 fatty acids**, the kind found in fish oil capsules, at approximately 1,000 milligrams per day. They are known to reduce the formation of blood clots and lower triglyceride levels. Look for supplements that provide the fatty acids EPA and DHA. *Tip:* Keep them in the freezer to avoid the unpleasant aftertaste.

24. **Add mineral supplements**: magnesium, 300 milligrams; calcium, 800 milligrams; and potassium.

    - Supplement your diet with antioxidants:
    - Vitamin E, 400 to 800 IUs (mixed tocopherols)
    - Vitamin C, 1000 milligrams (esterized is best)
    - Beta carotene, 6 milligrams
    - Selenium, 200 micrograms

If you are still struggling with cholesterol after making these lifestyle changes, there are medical options available. Most notably are the statin drugs, such as Crestor, Mevacor, Lipitor, Lescol, Pravachol, and Zocor. These drugs are the first line of treatment for most people with high cholesterol. These medications work best when combined with lifetime wellness lifestyle modifications.

Side effects of these medications can include intestinal problems, liver damage, and (in a few people) muscle tenderness. You should avoid taking other cholesterol-lowering drugs and anticoagulants (blood thinners). Also, you should avoid grapefruit juice and limit fresh grapefruit consumption while taking cholesterol-lowering drugs, as grapefruit can interfere with the liver's ability to metabolize these medications.

Get REAL Note: Statins block the production of cholesterol in the liver itself. They lower LDL ("bad" cholesterol) and triglycerides, and they have a mild effect in raising HDL ("good" cholesterol).

Use the knowledge you have available to you to maintain and improve your lifetime wellness lifestyle. Don't let things you cannot control burden you. Remember—focus on the outcomes that you want and not on the symptoms that you don't want. Maintaining your health is a lifelong project and one that requires your enthusiasm and attention. Be sure to give this aspect of wellness as much emphasis as all the rest. It can be the ticket to extend your wonderful and influential life. Those who love you will thank you.

Recommended Health Screenings Schedule

> **Get REAL Note:** Recommendations may vary among practitioners. This is a compilation based on multiple sources at the time of publication.

Immunizations

Influenza vaccinations: Annually if at high risk (the very young, the elderly, health or school workers, and the immune compromised).

Tetanus booster: Every ten years.

Pneumonia vaccination: One time after age 65, or sooner for those meeting high-risk criteria.

HPV vaccination: Series of three shots for girls ages 11 to 26.

Meningococcal vaccine: One time after Age 11 thru college years.

General Screenings

Annual physical exam: Includes blood pressure screening, pelvic exam, breast exam, digital rectal exam, and routine blood work. Note and track any unusual symptoms or changes. Bring a list of current medications, supplements and any questions you have.

Thyroid screening: Every five years for those age 35 and older or if symptomatic.

Blood glucose (for diabetes): Every three years for those age 45 and older or if symptomatic.

Bone density:

- Women—Baseline testing recommended at menopause.

- Men—At age 65.
- All—As directed by your doctor for predisposing conditions.

Vision screening:

- School age—As directed per school and physician.
- Ages 20 to 39—Baseline and as needed.
- Ages 40 to 64—Every two to four years.
- Ages 65 and older, or anyone having eye strain or difficulty reading smaller print—Every one to two years.

Glaucoma screening: Every five years or if symptomatic.

Dental checkup: Every six months and as needed for problems.

Hearing test: If experiencing difficulty in hearing certain words clearly.

Cardiovascular risk evaluation:

- Annual health history and physical.
- Total cholesterol and HDL (lipid panel)—Every five years, or yearly if history of abnormal results, hypertension, or other risk factors.

Cancer Risk Evaluation

Skin examination (American Cancer Society recommendations):

- Every three years for people between 20 and 40 years of age.
- Yearly for people age 40 and older.
- Yearly if numerous moles or history of abnormal skin cells.

Colon screening (American Cancer Society recommendations): Individuals over age 50 should have the following screenings.

- Fecal occult blood test—yearly.
- Flexible sigmoidoscopy—every five years.
- Colonoscopy—every ten years.
- Double contrast barium enema—every five to ten years.
- Additional screening as needed if symptomatic.

You should have colorectal cancer screening earlier and/or more often if you have any of the following colorectal cancer risk factors:

- Strong family history of colorectal cancer or polyps (cancer or polyps in a first-degree relative younger than 60 or in two first-degree relatives of any age).
- Families with hereditary colorectal cancer syndromes (familial adenomatous polyposis or hereditary non-polyposis colon cancer).
- A personal history of colorectal cancer or adenomatous polyps.
- A personal history of chronic inflammatory bowel disease.

Gender Specific Cancer Evaluation
Women age 40 to 50:

(Due to increased debate, discuss your personal breast and cervical cancer screening options with your physician.)

- Clinical breast exam (CBE)—Annually
- Mammogram—Annually after age 40 (baseline age 35).
- PAP test—Annually. (Testing every other year is acceptable in women who have had at least three normal annual PAP tests and

no history of an abnormal tests.) PAP tests help to detect cervical cancer risks.

Men age 40 to 50:

- Prostate screening—The American Cancer Society recommends annual prostate specific antigen (PSA) blood testing and digital rectal exams (DRE) of the prostate gland beginning at age 50. Men who are in high-risk groups, such as African Americans or men who have a history of prostate cancer in close family members, should talk with their health care providers about beginning screenings at a younger age.

Get REAL Bottom Line: Give yourself the gift of prevention! Schedule annual screenings around your birthday to always remember when they are due. Do your part to detect and prevent negative health issues. Early detection saves lives!

Get REAL Lifetime Wellness Prescription

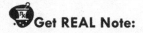**Get REAL Note:** Life has numerous variables. Often there is too much emphasis put on the "big two": nutrition and exercise. They are important, but there is much more that can be done to improve total wellness. Be open to new ideas and discover all the areas that can affect how you look and feel. Consider the following as a supplemental *lifestyle prescription* for good health.

- **Drink enough water daily.** Think about running your car without enough oil—that is a picture of your body without enough water. **Why?**—Your body depends on water to keep cells and body systems running smoothly. Water is also used to maintain blood volume, which is imperative for regulating body temperature and delivering oxygen and nutrients to the rest of the body. Water provides a medium for the biochemical reactions that occur at the cellular level. It is also crucial for the removal of waste products through the formation of urine by the kidneys. Your body cannot function at its optimum without adequate water consumption.

  A simple equation to help adults calculate their fluid needs is that for every pound of body weight, you need about half an ounce of fluid intake per day. For example, if you weigh 140 pounds, simply divide 140 by 2 to estimate your daily fluid needs in ounces (140 ÷ 2 = 70 ounces). Then divide by eight to estimate your fluid needs in cups per day, rounding up to the nearest full cup (70 ÷ 8 = 9 cups of fluid per day).

- **Take your vitamins.** Talk with your doctor about developing a proper nutritional supplement regime based on your personal needs and conditions. **Why?**—It is safe to say that most people do not meet their total nutritional needs through food alone. Taking vitamin and mineral supplements can help fill in the gaps. It is best to get these nutrients from food, but when that does not happen, supplements are a good alternative. Taken regularly, they can greatly improve daily functioning.

- **Don't ignore mental health.** Seek professional help for any persistent sadness or underlying depression. **Why?**—Your entire existence is affected by your mental health. If you have an imbalance in the brain that causes depression, you should seek professional help. A combination of medication and behavioral therapies could make a major difference in your life.

- **Read, study or listen to motivational messages routinely.** The mind needs to be renewed daily to stay in proper focus. **Why?**—Your thinking directly affects what you do. That makes it vitally important that you regularly are filling your mind with stimulating and uplifting information. Without it, you are more likely to lose focus and direction. Set your mind in a positive direction by purposefully seeking out inspirational messages on a routine basis.

- **Get adequate rest.** Seven to nine hours of sleep each night is recommended. **Why?**—It is at night that the body renews itself on a cellular level. You need adequate rest to ensure proper body functioning. It is the equivalent of charging your batteries. *Note:* You only have twenty-four hours to make up for any sleep deficits during that period of time.

- **Establish a relaxing bedtime routine.** Create a set of regular behaviors that will signal your body it is time for sleep. **Why?**—Your body becomes accustomed to repetitive patterns. When you actively take steps to create a relaxing routine, your body will respond to the association.

- **Dim the lights before bed.** Turn the lights down low and reduce stimulation during the hour before you go to sleep. **Why?**—This has to do with your sleep-wake cycle. Darkness promotes better sleep, and light stimulates the body's wakefulness.

- **Journal before bed.** The technique should fit your style. You can write lists, notes, or paragraphs. **Why?**—Journaling can allow you to free your mind from the cares of the day. Focusing on things you are thankful for creates positive thoughts and images before resting.

- **Keep your sleep cycles regular.** Go to bed and wake up within one to two hours of the same time each day. **Why?**—Your circadian rhythm is easily disturbed. Keeping a regular schedule will promote better rest and increase energy.

- **Take care of your teeth.** Floss once and brush twice daily. **Why?**—This simple step reduces chronic inflammation, which can lead to numerous health problems. It is responsible for an increased risk of disease.

- **Use aromatherapy.** The mind creates positive associations with pleasant scents. Just think about baby lotion, coconut tanning oil, or the aroma of baking cookies to understand what I mean. Aromatherapy uses essential oils to promote feelings of improved well-being. **Why?**—This type of therapy acts on the central nervous system. It has been known to relieve depression and anxiety, reduce stress, and restore both physical and emotional well-being. It can relax, uplift, sedate, or stimulate you. Aromatherapy using essential oils can help ease aches, pains, and injuries while relieving the discomforts of many health problems. Check into this time-honored therapy if you are new to its use.

- **Turn on the music.** Use music to awaken your senses and create positive associations **Why?**—Music affects the body in many health-promoting ways, which is the basis for music therapy. You can use music in your daily life and achieve many stress relief benefits on your own. One of the great benefits of music as a stress reliever is that it can be used while you conduct your regular activities. It can help you find increased enjoyment in your tasks and reduce stress from your day. Music creates associations in the mind. You suddenly remember that certain event when you hear a familiar song played. Your mind has created a link to the event, anchored in the song you heard there.

- **Increase your circle of friends.** Devote time to social pursuits and building relationships. **Why?**—Studies show that people who actively socialize and develop genuine friendships are happier and live longer. That's enough for me! Keeping that part of the brain stimulated seems to have positive benefits to overall health.

- **Focus on helping others.** Actively look for ways to help others on a regular basis. **Why?**—Helping others feels good, and it takes the mind off its own wants. Powerful brain chemicals are released when we help others. Besides, as Zig Ziglar always said, "You can get anything you want in life, if you help enough other people get what they want."

- **Place value on special events and milestones.** This includes those of friends and family along with your own. Attend events, send cards, and celebrate. Don't let those moments pass you by. **Why?**—Often when you look back on life, the things that seemed little at the time were really the big things. Remembering these special moments and commemorating them builds lifelong bonds with those you share them with. Just ask the girl who had her first baby shower.

PART VI

CREATING YOUR PLAN

CHAPTER 10

My Get REAL Wellness Plan

You have been introduced to the twenty Get REAL Concepts. Now it is time to create your Personal Wellness Plan. This chapter includes planning sheets for you to insert your personal goals and information. You can take the concepts provided in this guide and decide how they apply to you and your unique lifestyle.

As you insert your personal information into the planning sheets, you will be building your own Personal Wellness Plan (part of the Get REAL Fitness Plan). It will provide the framework for your goals and help you establish your own personal boundaries. Along with providing an outline, it also provides positive affirmations and personal accountability, designed to reinforce what you hope to achieve and how you plan to achieve it.

As time passes, it is easy to lose sight of your intended goals. When you need to gain perspective, you can reread the Personal Wellness Plan that you created. It should help you refocus and get back on track. Often as time passes you lose the sharp commitment you had to make those small changes. Over time these seemingly small choices can totally sabotage your intended goals. Self-evaluate weekly.

Get REAL Point:	It is the daily choices you make that will ultimately shape the success of your overall plan.

It is vital to regularly renew your mind and recall why you wanted to change in the first place. It is helpful to reread your plan daily until it becomes routine. Your Personal Wellness Plan serves as a reminder of how you felt that the Get REAL Concepts would work in your unique life. The outline provides affirmation of what you chose to do and gives you a reference for accountability. You will now create your Get REAL Fitness Plan and Personal Wellness Plan.

The Ten-Step Get REAL Fitness Plan

1. Using the Reality Check Measurements chart, take your measurements and record the results. Set realistic goals for each area and record them beside your current numbers. Complete that chart. Take a before photo in a body skimming layer or swimsuit. Include front, back and side view.

2. Choose any fitness testing (body fat percentage, step test, sit and reach flexibility) that will provide beneficial information for your personal plan. Determine your body mass index (BMI) based on the chart provided. Set your goal. Insert the results of that information into your Current Fitness Levels chart. Complete that chart. The tests are detailed in Appendix B.

3. Determine your maximum heart rate, resting heart rate, and target heart rate ranges. These numbers will help you to gauge the intensity of your workouts and see progress. Record the time it takes for you to complete one mile (1MT) and record your heart rate at the completion (HRR1) and after one, two and five minutes of rest (HRR2). Record all on the Cardio Tracking Log.

4. Choose an option from the Get REAL Cardiovascular Training Menu.

5. Choose an option from the Get REAL Resistance Training Menu.

6. Create an exercise incorporation plan based on your schedule and chosen options. Plan a goal week on the My Daily Schedule chart. Record actual daily events each evening.

7. Choose a nutrition strategy from the four options presented. Consider your calorie budget and fill out the corresponding

forms. Plan meals and shopping based on that. Remember: *Proper prior purposeful planning prevents poor performance!*

8. Complete your Personal Wellness Plan based on your choices. Use the Weekly Wellness Plan Self-Evaluation to help monitor your progress.

9. Create a weekly action plan to target challenging tasks. Fill out the My Get REAL Action Plan chart. Use the Get REAL Problem Solving worksheet to overcome obstacles.

10. Schedule your annual health screenings as needed for your age and health history risk factors. Record on the My Annual Screenings chart. Complete that chart.

Reality Check Measurements

Date_____

My Current Measurements   **My Goals**

Height: _____

Weight: _____   _____

(Upon awakening, after using bathroom)

Arms: _____   _____

(Mid-upper arm, largest part)

Bust: _____   _____

(Mid-breast, fullest part)

Thighs: _____   _____

(Widest part, below rise)

Calves: _____   _____

(Fullest part of lower leg)

Waist: _____   _____

(Narrowest area of the torso, keep loose)

Hips: _____   _____

(Widest part of hips or buttocks)

Waist-to-hip ratio: _____   _____

(Waist measurement divided by hip measurement)

Body fat percentage: _____%   Weight at goal %_____

Current Fitness Levels

(Results worksheet, see Appendix B for each test)

Date_____

WAIST TO HIP RATIO: ____

RISK: None____ Increased____ High____
Very High____ Extremely High____

Male=greater than 1.0 **Female**=greater than 0.8 **Pass/Fail**

BODY COMPOSITION: **BMI:** _____

RISK: Underweight____ Normal____ Overweight____
Obese____ Extremely Obese____

BODY FAT Percentage: ____

SIT AND REACH FLEXIBILITY: (Low Back/ Hamstrings)

_____Inches	Excellent	_____
	Good	_____
	Above Average	_____
	Average	_____
	Below Average	_____
	Poor	_____
	Very Poor	_____

THREE MINUTE STEP TEST: (Cardiovascular)

_____One Minute Heart Rate Recovery (HRR2)

_____Two Minute   Excellent   _____

_____Five Minute   Good   _____

                           Above Average   _____

                           Average   _____

                           Below Average   _____

                           Poor   _____

                           Very Poor   _____

Get REAL Note: A heart rate that recovers quickly is a mark of good health. Your heart rate should return to its pre-exercise level within ten to fifteen minutes after stopping exercise. Abnormal heart rate recovery is usually a sign that you are out of shape or deconditioned, but it could also represent a more serious heart condition. Check with your doctor before proceeding.

Cardio Tracking Log

- Maximal Heart Rate (220 minus your age)_____

- Resting Heart Rate_____

- Heart Rate Reserve (maximal minus resting rate) _____

- Low End of Target Heart Rate:

- (Heart Rate Reserve $\times$ 0.65) + (Resting Heart Rate) = _____

- High End of Target Heart Rate:

- (Heart Rate Reserve $\times$ 0.85) + (Resting Heart Rate) = _____

My Target Heart Rate Range is: _____– _____

Distance and Heart Rate Tracking

- One Mile Time (1MT) = _____

- Timed Distance (TD) = _____

- Heart Rate at Completion (HR1) = _____

- Completion Heart Rate Recovery (HRR2)

- After **one, two,** and **five** minutes of rest = ____ /____ /____

- For the following assessment, look at your **two-minute** HRR2:

____Normal HRR2 decrease of 15 to 25 beats per minute

____Abnormal HRR2 decrease of 12 or fewer beats per minute

Get REAL Cardiovascular Training Menu

#1 Beginner Cardiovascular and Aerobic Activity

Week	Suggested Total Minutes	Possibilities
One	40 min.	10 min./day for 4 days
Two	50 min.	10 min./day for 5 days
Three	60 min.	10 min./day for 6 days
Four	80 min.	20 min./day for 4 days
Five	100 min.	20 min./day for 5 days
Six	120 min.	30 min./day for 4 days

(Can be achieved in 5-minute increments)

#2 Moderate Cardiovascular and Aerobic Activity

Week	Suggested Total Minutes	Possibilities
One	80 min.	20 min./day for 4 days
Two	120 min.	30 min./day for 4 days
Three	160 min.	40 min./day for 4 days
Four	200 min.	40 min./day for 5 days
Five	225 min.	45 min./day for 5 days
Six	270 min.	45 min./day for 6 days

#3 Weight Loss Cardiovascular and Aerobic Activity

In Training (Conditioning Phase)

Week	Suggested Total Minutes	Possibilities
One	120 min.	30 min./day for 4 days
Two	160 min.	40 min./day for 4 days
Three	200 min.	50 min./day for 4 days
Four	250 min.	50 min./day for 5 days
Five	300 min.	50 min./day for 6 days
Six	360 min.	60 min./day for 6 days
Seven Plus	420 min.	60 min./day for 7 days

Get REAL Resistance Training Menu

Get REAL Exercise Option 1—All In One Day

Or choose to take one different area each day (Daily Option):
>
> CHEST
> SHOULDERS
> TRICEPS
> BICEPS
> BACK
> ABDOMINALS
> LEGS, HIPS, & BUTTOCKS
> CALVES

Get REAL Exercise Option 2—Two-Day Split

Day 1:

>
> CHEST
> SHOULDERS
> TRICEPS
> BICEPS
> BACK
> ABS

Day 2:

>
> LEGS, HIPS, & BUTTOCKS
> CALVES

Get REAL Exercise Option 3—Three-Day Split

Day 1:

CHEST
SHOULDERS
TRICEPS

Day 2:

LEGS, HIPS, & BUTTOCKS
CALVES

Day 3:

ABS
BACK
BICEPS

❖ Specific exercises are listed in Appendix E

My Daily Schedule

Month:_____

Sample Activity Log Key

A simple key can help you utilize space and visually see your exercise incorporation. Be sure to note the time spent. Tally your totals weekly to see your progress and to provide accountability. You can also jot notes and plan on the same calendar.

> **RT** (resistance training)
> **C** (cardio)
> **SF** (stretch and flexibility exercise)
> **TD** (timed distance)
> **PRT** (personal relaxation time)
> **1MT** (one-mile time)
> **HR1** (heart rate at completion of TD)
> **HRR2** (heart rate after $\underline{x}$ minutes of rest)

Get REAL Nutrition Strategies

Developing an effective nutrition strategy to meet your personal needs is essential. You can use one of the four following strategies to incorporate *realistic* and *healthy* nutrition into your personal wellness plan. The options are the *Budgeting Method, Plate Method, Carbohydrate Sensitive Method,* and *Calorie Shifting Method.* Choose your strategy based on what will work best for you and your lifestyle. It must be a style of eating that you can commit to following as part of your lifestyle, not just as a temporary diet.

Get REAL Nutrition Option 1: Budgeting Method

With this option, you choose a calorie range, then plan and track your intake using the recommended servings for that calorie range. This method helps you approximate the right serving size by using your hand and eyes to visualize the size of a healthy portion.

> **Get REAL Note:** It is not necessary to do math at every meal! That would not be realistic for most people. But you can develop an "eye" for portions using this "handy" reference guide.

- **Protein** = size of the palm of your hand
- **Carbohydrates** = size of your fist
- **Favorable carbs** (higher fiber or low glycemic index) = two loose fists (low glycemic carbs break down slowly during digestion and delay the release of sugar into the bloodstream)
- **Unfavorable carbs** (very starchy or high glycemic index) = one tight fist (high glycemic carbs break down quickly during digestion and release sugar rapidly into the bloodstream)

Protein

A portion of protein is equal to the size and thickness of your palm. (Other references compare a serving to a deck of cards or a checkbook.) Your hand can be a good guideline to determine healthy portions. It is relative to the size of your body and therefore your protein needs.

Protein sources other than meat, poultry, or fish include:

Eggs (1 egg)

Beans (1/2 cup)   Tofu (1/2 cup)

Peanut butter (1½–2 Tbsp.)   Dairy (½–1 cup)

Carbohydrates

Portions of carbohydrates can be judged by the size of your fist. Carbohydrates are classified as either *favorable* or *unfavorable.*

➢ If you choose *favorable* carbohydrates, two big, loose fist's worth equal one serving.

➢ If you choose *unfavorable* carbohydrates, you get only one tight fist's worth to equal one serving.

Favorable carbohydrates (also known as complex carbohydrates) have higher fiber content and lower glycemic index. Fiber allows food to be digested more slowly, which sustains blood sugar and reduces hunger. Fiber also helps maintain proper digestion and regulate waste elimination. Note that favorable carbohydrates are especially helpful and important for carb-sensitive or insulin-resistant people.

Favorable carbohydrates include:

- **Whole grains** (grains higher in fiber content), including long-grain, wild, and brown rice.
- **Legumes** such as beans and lentils.
- **Vegetables** such as squash, carrots, onions, sweet potatoes, and canned pumpkin.
- **Low-glycemic fruits** such as apples, berries, melons, cherries, grapefruit, kiwi, lemons, limes, oranges, peaches, pears, pineapple, plums, strawberries, and fruit and vegetable juices.

Unfavorable carbohydrates are not "bad" foods. They just serve a different function in the body, and you require less of them. They have lower fiber content and a higher glycemic index. These foods are burned up quickly by the body and spike the blood sugar. Note that these can cause trouble for carb-sensitive or insulin-resistant people.

Unfavorable carbohydrates include:

- **Simple sugars and highly processed foods** like desserts and sweets. These are also known as quick carbohydrates or fast-acting sugars (the "carbage").
- **Highly refined grains** (lower in fiber content) like regular pasta, white breads, and white rice.
- **Starchy vegetables** like potatoes, peas and corn.
- **High-glycemic fruits** like bananas, figs, prunes, raisins, and grapes.

> **Get REAL Point:** Eating too many unfavorable carbohydrates can cause mood swings, tiredness, cravings, and weight gain.

Dietary Fat

A little goes a long way when it comes to portions of dietary fat. Most people do not need to add fats to their diet. The main factor is seeking healthy fats and decreasing unhealthy sources. Learning to eat some healthy fats and combining them with your other food choices becomes the big challenge. The other factor concerns your mindset. You must allow yourself to eat fat without feeling guilty.

This guilt often holds people in bondage to overindulgence. Often people try very hard to be "good" in an attempt to follow these low-fat diets. This restriction leads to frustration and eventual deviation from their original plan. When people deviate from a rigid plan, they often completely abandon any healthy living principles. Whatever good they did through their period of low-fat dieting is completely offset by the impending overindulgence that results from restriction and deprivation.

Fat in our diet serves a purpose. It signals the body to feel full and helps to balance blood sugar levels. The problem comes when people eat too much fat or get all their fat from unhealthy sources. It is very easy to overindulge in fatty foods. This is because of the abundance of highly processed fast food and convenience items we have.

I know people who won't eat nuts because of the fat in them. This is an example of the current mindset that keeps people from losing weight. Foods such as nuts contain healthy fat and are a good source of protein. They are a natural and whole food.

Balancing fat takes practice. It is easy to go overboard and eat too much. That is where problems will arise if you are not mindful in your eating. If your protein source is high in fat, don't add any extra dietary fat. Foods like olives, avocados, nuts, and olive oil are all wonderful natural fats that can enhance health and help balance eating.

Dairy is another healthy option that people often stay away from because of the fat content. Dairy products are full of nutrients that your body utilizes for daily functioning. They are a source of protein and healthy fats. Adding these foods back into your diet can help maintain improved food balance and help you stay on track.

> **Get REAL Note:** The budgeting method has its foundation in the diabetic exchange plan to help you determine calorie and nutritional values.

The exchange system works by grouping foods into six categories: bread/starch, meat/protein, vegetable, fruit, dairy and fat. Within each category, foods have a similar nutrient makeup, so little math is involved in meal planning. Any food from a certain category can be exchanged for another in that category, since they are similar in the amount of carbohydrate, calories, fat, and protein. Note that serving sizes may vary from item to item.

The following chart shows the amounts of nutrients in one serving from each exchange list. You can use this information for meal planning. It will help you to more accurately determine the calorie values of the foods you are eating. It is a valuable tool in learning about portion control and the nutrient value of the foods you are consuming. It also aids in understanding meal balancing.

> **Get REAL Tip:** For detailed exchange lists, you can do a Web search for *diabetic exchange lists*.

Food Exchange List	Carbohydrate (grams)	Protein (grams)	Fat (grams)	Calories
I. Bread/Starch	15	3	trace	80
II. Meat/Protein	(See fat content below for details)			
Very Lean	.	7	0–1	35
Lean	.	7	3	55
Medium-Fat	.	7	5	75
High-Fat	.	7	8	100
III. Vegetables	5	2	.	25
IV. Fruit	15	.	.	60
V. Dairy	(See fat content below for details)			
Skim	12	8	0–3	90
Low-fat	12	8	5	120
Whole	12	8	8	150
VI. Fat	.	.	5	45

Get REAL Tip:	Strive to not let more than three to four hours pass without some form of balanced eating. The five fingers of your hand can remind you to eat at least five times a day—three meals and two snacks, or five similarly proportioned eating episodes. This will depend on your personal style. Remember, snacks can also be the liquid calories in juice or milk.

Get REAL Nutrition Option 2: Plate Method

This approach teaches you how to fill your plate in healthy proportions. By using this simple method, you can go anywhere and choose meals with confidence.

- ✓ Divide your plate in half.
- ✓ Fill the lower half with your fruits and nonstarchy vegetables.
- ✓ Divide the top half again.
- ✓ Fill one side with your palm-size amount of protein.
- ✓ Fill the other side with your starchy carbohydrate item.

Eat one plate, three times a day, plus two small snacks.

- ✓ Your snack should be balanced, with a protein source and between 100 and 300 calories.
- ✓ When you eat a fast-acting carbohydrate or sugar, always balance it with a protein source, complex carb, or healthy fat.
- ✓ Pick up no other munchies, because they can stimulate hunger.
- ✓ Avoid liquid calories, or count them in as part of your meal.

If you eat a simple or unfavorable carbohydrate, *always* pair it with a protein, complex carbohydrate, or healthy fat. This will keep your blood sugar stable and avoid spikes and crashes in your energy level. It also greatly reduces cravings for sugar and keeps you full longer!

A solid eating plan will balance the ratio of carbohydrates with your proteins and fats. Ideally, you will eat a slightly greater percentage of carbohydrates, but you must also closely balance that with your amounts of protein and fats at *each* eating opportunity. Remember the (P2B) ratio: 7 grams of protein to balance every 15 grams of carbs, at each eating episode.

151

> **Get REAL Tip:** P2B requires planning on your part, so recall our mantra: Proper prior purposeful planning prevents poor performance!

This style of eating should help reduce your cravings and allow you to sense true hunger and fullness signals. This can allow you to eat more sensibly at meals. Start changing the way you think about eating and how you combine your foods. It is all about providing gentle boundaries and giving yourself the ultimate freedom to work within that structure. This allows you to eat with intention instead of restriction. This approach works great for people who are not carb sensitive.

Get REAL Nutrition Option 3: Carb-Sensitive Method

Some people fall into a group dubbed as "carbohydrate sensitive," or CS for short. These people face very real chemical and hormonal changes upon eating carbohydrates. Often they are called "sugar addicts" because of this sensitivity. For CS people, one bite of a simple carbohydrate sets off a series of real reactions in the body. In a nutshell, the carb consumption increases hunger and decreases the sense of fullness that non-CS people feel. It actually produces a compulsion to eat.

Eating carbs initially produces a pleasurable feeling by activating pleasure centers in the brain. But this is followed by an uneasy feeling, weariness, and an urge to snack more due to the body's attempt to recreate the pleasurable feeling. For some unknown reason, CS people accumulate an excess of insulin that signals the body to conserve energy. They actually become hungrier with each carb-rich meal or snack they consume. The body will then begin to store the excess insulin in the form of fat.

> **Get REAL Note:** For CS people, the carbohydrate-insulin/carbohydrate-serotonin connection has malfunctioned. That connection is the basis for Nutrition Option 3.

Have you ever wondered how some people seem to have such restraint? They can eat a little bit of some tasty dish and then feel full and push away from the table. If you are like me, this seems like some kind of magical witchcraft! But in reality, it is less magical, more chemical. Brain chemistry is affected when signals are not sent and received normally.

For CS people, serotonin levels do not rise sufficiently. As a result, the feeling of being satisfied is never delivered. This leads the CS person to overeat and begins a cycle of craving more carbohydrates. The constant "needing something more" feeling can never quite be squelched. This contributes to weight gain and continued feelings of hunger.

The production of insulin will continue to rise with each subsequent consumption of carbohydrates. Larger quantities of carbs may be consumed more frequently without any increase in satisfaction. For people facing this situation, food becomes the enemy. They become frustrated with their efforts and this can lead to feelings of self loathing for not being able to control hunger. Often they would rather not eat at all than start to eat and then not want to stop.

> **Get REAL Note:** The body burns carbohydrates for energy. Take in more than you can burn, and it will be stored as fat.

Eating numerous high-carbohydrate foods by themselves often leads people to feel unsatisfied. Much of this has to do with blood sugar. Carbohydrates will spike your blood sugar, giving you a temporary boost.

153

What goes up must come down, though, and that means the fast spike will result in a fast crash.

When we are feeling low and sluggish from a sugar crash, what do we crave? We tend to crave more carbohydrates or sugars to recreate the high. This causes a cycle of mood swings and overindulgence.

Carbohydrates stimulate insulin secretion. Insulin is the body's means of lowing blood sugar. Too much insulin causes you to crave more carbs in an attempt to elevate blood sugar to a therapeutic level. Insulin turns excess carbohydrates into fat! By monitoring carbohydrate consumption, you can better control your insulin production. Maintaining insulin at a balanced level improves your ability to burn excess body fat.

Whether what you just ate will be used for immediate energy or stored as body fat depends on the timing and amount of your intake. Dietary fat and protein, on the other hand, do not stimulate insulin secretion. Protein is an important component in any eating plan. Your body uses protein for essential daily functioning. It helps you build muscle and sustains your blood sugar and insulin levels. Protein consumption can reduce your cravings and increase fullness.

The body releases insulin in two phases:

- **The preload phase** begins within minutes of eating carbohydrates. During this phase, the pancreas releases a fixed amount of insulin, no matter how many carbs are consumed. This is determined by the amount of carbs consumed in earlier meals.

- **The second phase** takes place about seventy-five to ninety minutes after eating. It is dependent on the number of carbs consumed during that eating episode. The body recognizes whether the first phase was sufficient to handle the current consumption. It will adjust insulin production to meet the current need.

CS people tend to sustain a higher insulin level in the blood. The reason for this is not fully understood. It seems to coincide with a decreased number and sensitivity of insulin receptor sites. Too much insulin in the blood for too long causes the cells to change in such a way that less insulin is able to enter, and there is a decrease in the actual number of receptor sites. Subsequently, this causes your body to stop responding to insulin (insulin resistance) and instead grab every calorie it can and deposit it as fat.

This insulin-resistant state means that no matter how little you eat, you will gradually gain weight. At the same time, your cells cannot absorb the glucose they need, so they signal your brain that you need more carbohydrates or sugars. The result is persistent food cravings. The challenge is to determine whether you are carbohydrate sensitive.

Common CS symptoms:

- ✓ You feel tired or fatigued in the middle of the day.
- ✓ You start to have cravings during midafternoon, between lunch and dinner.
- ✓ You crave sweets about an hour or two after eating a full meal, including dessert.
- ✓ You find it more difficult to control eating after a carb-rich breakfast than after having only coffee or nothing at all.
- ✓ You find it is easier to not eat most of the day than to eat small meals throughout the day.
- ✓ You find it hard to stop eating sweets, starches, or snack foods once you start.
- ✓ You often feel like you could eat another whole meal after you have just finished one.
- ✓ When feeling down, a sugary snack makes you feel better.

✓ If potatoes, bread, pasta, or dessert are offered, you often skip the vegetables and salad.

✓ You become sleepy and lethargic after a large, starchy meal.

✓ You experience unexplained feelings of anxiety or anger.

✓ You have an unusually heightened emotional state.

These are just a few of the things that many CS people experience. If you relate to only a few of them, then it is likely not CS. But if almost every one of these characteristics seems like you, there is a good chance CS is the problem. For you, eating three average meals and two snacks with unbalanced carbs can cause more harm than good. It would constantly trigger your insulin load to be activated, making you feel hungry all the time and never satisfied.

If you are carb sensitive, you need to eat in a way that stops the cycle of excess insulin production. When carbs are eaten less frequently, less insulin will be produced. The body will have a decreased tendency to store the excess calories in its fat cells and will be more capable of breaking down stored fat.

Get REAL Point: Carbohydrate sensitivity seems to have two main issues: the *frequency* and *duration* of carbohydrate eating episodes.

Consuming carbohydrates during a limited period of time appears to decrease the usual overproduction of insulin. When carbs are consumed within a single hour, the CS person experiences less hunger. This is because of the body's limited ability to produce insulin at any one time. If the consumption time is limited, the insulin production time is too. This allows the body to break the excess insulin cycle.

CS Eating Solution A: Low-Carb

- Eat two low-carb (LC) meals daily. (Carbs trigger cravings, remember?) Forgo any food or beverage that contains more than 4 grams of carbs per serving. Save fruit for your other meal.

- Eat one "anything goes" (AG) meal daily. (Really—anything!) Remember, be sensible and don't binge. Allow yourself those carbs you have been craving, while also rounding out your daily nutritional needs.

> **Get REAL Note:** The AG meal must be consumed within sixty consecutive minutes to avoid the excess insulin production cycle.

- Whatever meal you choose for your AG meal, it should consistently stay at the same time of day. The meals could occasionally be switched for special occasions, but then go back to your normal meal times.

- Have one LC snack. Forgo any food or beverage that contains more than 4 grams of carbs per serving. Save fruit for your AG meal.

If you are carb sensitive, this way of eating will help you control your constant cravings without feeling deprived. You will have to be disciplined for two meals. With a little planning, you can do it! You have the AG meal to keep you from feeling deprived.

Remember, you are human—you will have deviations from your plan. Make a point of getting back to your routine as soon as you can, always keeping in mind that your cravings are directly related to your last carb consumption. Give yourself an advantage. Eat to control your CS food feelings.

CS Eating Solution B: Pair-to-Balance (P2B)

No matter how effective a plan is, if you won't stick to it, it is worthless. If Solution A seems too restrictive or too difficult to maintain in your REAL situation, I recommend a kinder, softer version. Keeping in mind the goal of controlling cravings caused by a hyperinsulin state, you will use protein to balance meals.

1. Eat a breakfast that includes a balanced protein serving.

2. Eat at least three regularly timed meals with a balanced protein serving (maintain as close to regularly timed as possible, with three to four hours in between).

3. Choose a protein snack or protein/complex carbohydrate combination snack. You have the option to either snack or not snack—just maintain the idea of a balanced protein serving every three to four hours. Plan to have available sources on hand.

4. Consider your P2B ratio (7 grams protein to balance 15 grams of carbs).

Don't think of this as a high-protein plan. It is an adequate protein plan. Most CS people do not get enough protein in their natural diet. They tend to not choose those sources when given starchy or sugary options.

Mindful addition of protein to each eating episode is a great place to start. Be extremely cautious of eating a sweet treat alone. This will seem pleasurable at first, but remember that you are carb-sensitive and realize the destructive journey it will lead you on.

Save sweet treats to consume with your meal. Remember, you can eat them—just think about when to eat them and what to eat them with so that you do not begin the cascading spiral of craving and pleasure-food seeking. Understanding how you react differently to carb consumption will make choosing food combinations less difficult and easier to accept. There is REAL chemistry behind those cravings!

CS "Go-To" Snacks and Add-Ins:

- Nuts (any)
- Cheese sticks
- Eggs—hard boiled
- Cottage cheese
- Peanut butter and whole wheat crackers
- Ham/cream cheese rollups
- Meat rollups using low-carb wraps
- Cheese and whole wheat crackers
- V-8 juice
- Meat and cheese on whole wheat crackers
- Protein shakes or bars
- Yogurt
- Peanut butter and apple slices
- Summer sausage
- Milk
- Peanut butter, raisins, and celery
- Beef jerky
- Meat sticks
- Tuna
- Chicken chunks
- Nonstarchy vegetables
- Flax meal (ground flaxseed) as an add-in

Get REAL Nutrition Option 4: Calorie Shifting

Your body is smart and can quickly become accustomed or adapted to consistent patterns. This option is based on the body's adaptation principle. It keeps your metabolism guessing and helps it run more efficiently. Calorie shifting is a good tool to use when you hit a plateau or your weight loss has stagnated. It is designed to give a good diet an edge, but doesn't work well if your current diet is poor.

Calorie shifting works by providing a formula you can apply to any plan of your choice. The theory is that if you consume X number of calories on your current diet, and have been consistently following it, your body will expect to receive approximately X number of calories every day. Your body adapts to this and begins to work less efficiently. Never choose a reduced calorie option for greater than seventy-two hours. This triggers fat storage in attempt to fight off starvation.

By altering your calorie intake, you keep your body guessing. This method can push your metabolism to work harder because it no longer knows what to expect. Calorie shifting can help reset a previously stalled metabolism. This formula works best for detail-oriented people. It is a fine-tuning method and can be applied to most eating styles. It would be used temporarily to move past a plateau.

Get REAL Calorie Shifting Example:

- **Establish a baseline.** You need to consistently follow your diet for at least a month. This brings your body to expect a regular intake of that amount of calories. In this example, the baseline is 2,000 calories.
- **Ramp up 300 calories.** Two times a week for the first week, add 300 calories to your diet. On Monday and Thursday, eat 2,300 calories.
- **Cut down 500 calories.** Two times a week for the second week, subtract 500 calories. On Tuesday and Friday, eat 1,500 calories.
- **Ramp up 400 calories.** Two times a week for the third week, add 400 calories to your diet. On Wednesday and Saturday, eat 2,400 calories.
- **Cut down 500 calories.** Two times a week for the fourth week, subtract 500 calories. On Thursday and Sunday, eat 1,500 calories.

Creating a Get REAL Calorie Budget

My Personal Calorie Range is: _____ – _____

Recommended Servings (per chart below)
_____ – _____ Bread/Starch
_____ – _____ Meat/Protein
_____ – _____ Vegetables
_____ – _____ Fruit
_____ – _____ Dairy
_____ – _____ Fat

Use this chart as a reminder of the number of servings you need from each food group to meet your daily caloric range.

My Calorie Range Choice and Servings Recommended

Calorie Levels with Suggested Number of Servings						
Calorie Levels	Bread/ Starch	Meat/ Protein	Vegetables	Fruit	Dairy	Fat
1200	5–6	4–5	3	2-3	2–3	3–4
1400	6–7	5–6	3–4	3–4	2–3	3–4
1500	7–8	5–6	3–4	3–4	2–3	3–4
1600	8–9	6–7	3–4	3–4	2–3	3–4
1800	10–11	6–7	3–4	3–4	2–3	4–5
2000	11–12	6–7	4–5	4–5	2–3	5–6
2200	12–13	7–8	4–5	4–5	2–3	6–7
2400	13–14	8–9	4–5	4–5	2–3	7–8
2600	14–15	9–10	5	5	2–3	7–8
2800	15–16	9–10	5	5	2–3	9–10

You can either monitor calories (just numbers) or line up your servings to match your calorie level. What you choose will depend on what works best for you and what you will continue doing. Using this chart keeps you mindful of healthy portions and balanced nutrition.

You may copy the following log and keep it with you.

Get REAL Accountability

Plan (How I would like to divide daily servings)

My Personal Calorie Range is: _____–_____ DATE_____

Recommended Servings	AM	Noon	PM	Snacks
____Breads/Starches	_____	_____	_____	_____
____Meats/Protein	_____	_____	_____	_____
____Vegetables	_____	_____	_____	_____
____Fruit	_____	_____	_____	_____
____Dairy	_____	_____	_____	_____
____Fat	_____	_____	_____	_____

What I Ate Today (Note Amount)

Breakfast:_____

Lunch:_____

Dinner:_____

Snacks:_____

Log (How I actually divided daily servings)

Make a mark for each serving consumed and when—use best estimate.

Recommended Servings	AM	Noon	PM	Snacks
_____Breads/Starches	_____	_____	_____	_____
_____Meats/Protein	_____	_____	_____	_____
_____Vegetables	_____	_____	_____	_____
_____Fruit	_____	_____	_____	_____
_____Dairy	_____	_____	_____	_____
_____Fat	_____	_____	_____	_____

Water: __ __ __ __ __ __ __ __

Vitamins and or supplements taken: _____ Yes _____ No

Personal relaxation time taken: _____ Yes _____ No

Comments: Note unusual events, challenges, or victories below.

My Weekly Grocery Planner

Breads/Starches (Carbs)

_____   _____

_____   _____

Meats/Fish/Eggs/Beans (Protein)

_____   _____

_____   _____

Vegetables

_____   _____

_____   _____

Fruits

_____   _____

_____   _____

_____   _____

Dairy

_____   _____

_____   _____

Fats

_____   _____

Processed/Packaged

_____   _____

_____   _____

_____   _____

Start looking at how you shop in a new way—Shop with purpose!
Note (F) for frozen section.

Personal Wellness Plan

- I am changing my attitude concerning health and fitness on

  _____ (date)

- I am making a commitment to consistent moderation in the areas of food intake, exercise, and personal relaxation time.

- I am making these changes because I want _____

  _____

  _____

- The things that matter most to me in life are

  _____   _____

  _____   _____

  _____   _____

- I say no to extra obligations that do not line up with the things that matter most to me.

- I commit to spend my time in a way that reflects what is important to me. To ensure this, I will regularly evaluate my schedule.

- My short-term goal is to _____

  _____

  by_____ (date)

- This is realistic and obtainable. I can do this!

- When I reach this goal, I will set a new short-term goal.

- My long-term goal is to _____

  _____

  by_____ (date)

- These goals can be adjusted as I choose.

- I regularly look outside myself and family, seeking ways to help others.

- I encourage someone daily (whether by note, card, e-mail, or in person).
- I make every effort to attend the special events of close friends and family.
- I regularly touch base with distant friends and close neighbors.
- I live in the moment. I am fully present in whatever situation I am in.
- I set aside time each day to pursue a personal interest or to just relax.
- I understand that not taking time for myself causes stress, leads to illness, and promotes poor habits.
- I can do everything required of me when I care for myself first.
- Some ways I will take time for myself, and some activities I enjoy, are:

  _____

  _____

  _____

- I have identified times and situations that often become problems.
- I do not let these areas of life sabotage my efforts or steal my time.
- When faced with _____

      I plan to _____

- When faced with _____

      I plan to _____

- When faced with _____

      I plan to _____

- When faced with _____

      I plan to _____

- I choose to eat mindfully and with purpose.
- The nutrition strategy I choose is _____

  _____

- My calorie budget range currently is ____ to ____ calories per day.
- I shift my calorie range if I hit a plateau or my needs change.

- I plan ahead daily to have what I will need on hand for each day.
- I do not make any food off-limits or label it a "bad" food.
- I can eat out, eat my favorite foods, and enjoy deserts, all in moderation.
- I no longer feel guilty about deviating from my plan.
- Deviation is normal, and I will choose to make better choices at the next available opportunity. (Guilt is an excuse used to keep bad habits.)
- I do not blame others or make excuses when I don't meet my goals.
- Because I am accountable for what I consume, I have the freedom to decide what is really important to me, and if I want something bad enough, to account for it.
- I look forward to doing the things I outline in my plan because I am in control of all my choices.
- The cardiovascular training plan I choose is _____
  _____

- I am going to rediscover my love of (activity, hobby, interest, or talent) _____
  _____
  _____

- I add small amounts of purposeful movement into each day.
- Some of the ways I will do this are by _____
  _____
  _____
  _____

- I realize that I reap the benefits of my purposeful new behaviors.
- I have chosen to exercise and will track my progress. I am consistent.
- I log the time I spend in physical activity until I am more comfortable with my new routine.

- Activities I enjoy that will raise my heart rate for greater than five minutes are _____

  _____

  _____

  _____

- I commit to spend _____ hours a week to the above activities.
- This amounts to _____ per day and is my exercise time budget.
- I am accountable to the budget I set for myself.
- I am mindful not to dump too much into one day.
- I guard against procrastination, because it enables excuses.
- I see how important resistance training is to overall good health.
- The resistance training plan I choose is _____

  _____

- I commit to spend _____ minutes/hours a week to toning and firming my muscles and strengthening my bones.
- I can break this time up however I choose during the week.
- I can alter my plan however I choose to meet my goal.
- I do not attempt too much, too soon.
- I start slow and progress my activity level gradually.
- I remember to vary my routine periodically to avoid adaptation.
- I regularly evaluate and revise my plan as needed.
- If I become bored or unhappy with my plan, I modify it.
- In the event I make choices that are not in line with my plan, I do not get discouraged and revert to old habits.
- I choose to make a better choice at the next opportunity.
- If discouraged, I call or e-mail _____ @

  _____

- This is *my* Personal Wellness Plan—with guidance, I choose what will work for me and my lifestyle.
- I am unique, and so are my responsibilities, my schedule, my personality, and what motivates me.
- I am ready to Get REAL and make changes to enhance my life.

_____   _____

(Signed)   (Date)

Get REAL Bottom Line: To be effective, you must review your plan regularly. Post it where you will be able to read it daily, or keep it with you so you can refer to it when you are falling victim to old habits.

Weekly Wellness Plan Self-Evaluation

Week _____ to _____	Yes	Usually	Not so much
I review my Personal Wellness Plan regularly.			
Daily decisions line up with my "What Matters Most" list.			
I have focused on living in the "now" and being mindful.			
I live with purpose and intention and practice thought reframing.			
I stayed on track with my nutrition strategy this week.			
I drank enough water this week.			
I added nutrition to my eating episodes.			
I was conscious of fruits, vegetables, and protein sources.			
I took my daily vitamins or supplements (as approved by my physician).			
I engaged in resistance training at least twice this week.			
I raised my heart rate for more than twenty minutes at least three times.			
I handled deviations with success.			
I managed my schedule, pruning unproductive activity.			
I took at least ten minutes for active relaxation daily.			
I took time daily for personal/spiritual enrichment.			
I spent time on a personal hobby.			
I sought support when I needed it.			
I kept my commitment to encouraging others.			
I spent time on building healthy relationships.			

Get REAL Action Planning

Creating an action plan can be extremely beneficial when targeting any behavior for change. It serves as a visual reminder to track progress and provide accountability for the change. Here are the main steps to create your action plan:

1. Determine what you want to do. This must be very specific, realistically achievable, and measurable.

2. Decide when or how much you are going to do it.

3. Choose how many days a week you are going to do it.

Be sure to specify something you can confidently achieve in a week's time. If you have a low level of confidence, you should alter the goal to make it more achievable. This should increase your confidence and the likelihood of achievement. If you can't meet your goal, it is easy to become discouraged. Goals can be worded in a variety of ways, depending on the type of goal chosen.

Examples of Get REAL Action Planning:

I will *(what)* walk around the block *(when)* after supper *(how many times)* three nights this week.

- Drink three glasses of water daily for at least five days.
- Walk twenty minutes three times before Saturday.
- Take my daily vitamins at least five days this week.
- Read a book for pleasure for ten minutes at least four times.
- Eat three different fruits or vegetables daily for five days.
- Set aside one date night this week.
- Strength train twice for ten minutes before Sunday.

Think of the top six things you would like to target. Create an action plan for each. Focus on only one action plan the first week, then continue to add a new one each week. Copy and post plans weekly or share them with someone. After six weeks, you should be on your way to six new healthy habits!

My Get REAL Action Plan

1. What do I want to do? _____

2. How often will I do this? _____

3. When will I do this? (Specific day or time) _____

4. To whom will I be accountable for this behavior and how?

_____

_____

Action Plan   Week #_____

I will_____

When_____

How many times_____

	Met Goal	N/A	Not So Much
Monday	_____	____	_____
Tuesday	_____	____	_____
Wednesday	_____	____	_____
Thursday	_____	____	_____
Friday	_____	____	_____
Saturday	_____	____	_____
Sunday	_____	____	_____

Action Plan   Week #_____

I will_____

When_____

How many times_____

	Met Goal	N/A	Not So Much
Monday	_____	____	_____
Tuesday	_____	____	_____
Wednesday	_____	____	_____
Thursday	_____	____	_____
Friday	_____	____	_____
Saturday	_____	____	_____
Sunday	_____	____	_____

Get REAL Problem Solving

When you are trying to change a behavior or create a new one, the first plan may not always be the most workable plan. You may need to try something else, modify your plan, or give yourself more time to reach your goal. Often, breaking the issue down into smaller, more doable steps can make the task easier to accomplish. Whatever the reason for not meeting your goals, a simple problem-solving technique can be very helpful in overcoming most barriers.

1. Identify the actual problem (very important).

2. List several possible ideas to solve the problem.

3. Select one method to try. (Try it for at least two weeks.)

4. Assess the results.

5. Substitute another idea if the first didn't work.

6. Utilize other resources, such as asking family, friends, or professionals for input and ideas.

7. If none of the ideas you try work accept that the problem may not be solvable at this time.

By following this sequence each time you are unable to reach your goal, you will be better equipped to find solutions to your barriers. This may seem overly simplistic, but it is very beneficial to write down the issues and brainstorm to find solutions. This method gives issues validity and encourages you to reach your goal.

To self-manage your behavior changes, you must:

1. Set goals.

2. Make a list of alternatives for reaching the goal.

3. Make short-term action plans weekly toward that goal.

4. Carry out your plan.

5. Check on your progress weekly.

6. Make midcourse changes as necessary.

7. Use rewards for a job well done.

Get REAL Bottom Line: By self-managing barriers to change, you can boost your confidence and chances of success. This method of problem solving provides a solid framework for you to use in any area of your life.

My Annual Screenings

(Advice will vary; check with your health care practitioner.)

Screening	Date	Doctor/Phone
Complete Physical Exam—Annually		
Routine Blood Work—Annually		
Thyroid Screening— Every five years (age 35 and up)		
Blood Glucose (for diabetes)— Every three years (age 45 and up)		
Vision Screening—Annually		
Dental Checkup— Every six months or annually		
Skin Cancer Screening—Annually		
Bone Density—Doctor guided		
Condition Specific Testing—If indicated		
Colon Cancer Screenings (age 50 and up):		
Fecal occult blood test—Annually		
Flexible Sigmoidoscopy—Every five years		
Colonoscopy— Every ten years		
Double contrast barium enema— Every five to ten years		
Women:		
Clinical Breast Exam—Annually		
Mammogram—Baseline age 35 (age 40 and up) —Annually		
Pap Smear—Annually or biannually		
Men:		
Prostate Screening (age 50 and up)— Annually		

PART VII

THE GET REAL SKINNY

CONCLUSION

Enjoying Where You Are, on the Way to Where You Are Going

Losing weight and getting healthier can feel like a huge battle. In a way it is. You are fighting old thought patterns and habits that have become comfortable, much like a default setting that you can achieve without much thought or effort. Here is a Get REAL breakdown to help you:

The Five Steps to Get REAL Change

- Have a strong desire for the change.
- Have a willingness to change.
- Have an ability to enact the change.
- Have a determination to do whatever it takes to achieve and maintain your goals.
- Have a resolve to not give up, even when it gets tough.

Without these five crucial factors, you will not fully achieve the results you envision. Many people want *Biggest Loser*-type results but don't want to put in the *Biggest Loser* kind of effort. This is a process, a journey, and not just a means to an end. Learn to love the process. Taking each moment as it comes reduces dread and improves results.

One of the most valuable lessons you can learn is to enjoy your life while you are working toward your goals. Part of that enjoyment comes from being fully present in each moment. The practice of mindfulness is an underutilized tactic. Mindfulness means you choose to fully focus on what is going on right now. In the guise of multitasking, people often fail to enjoy what they are doing due to dwelling on past or future events.

When you think about it, what is so stressing at this very moment? Most would say, "Nothing right now." Much of the anxiety and sadness that we encounter comes from past events or perceived future events. It has nothing to do with what is happening at this very moment.

Learning to harness the energy of the moment and choosing not to ruminate on past or future events can greatly improve your sense of well-being and peacefulness. This is a simple but powerful way of refocusing your attention to the here and now. When you allow your thoughts to dwell in the "what was" and the "what is yet to be," you waste valuable energy and expend emotions that would be better left conserved.

Too many people allow themselves to get wound up and stressed out over things that have happened or things that they think will happen. Allow your mind to fully focus on the present moment and experience the peace that comes with having your mind, body, and spirit fully in the current moment you are experiencing. For some, this will be a whole new way of approaching life.

You have the ability to harness your thoughts and control their direction. Mindfulness can be a gift you give yourself. Practicing it regularly allows you to become more at peace and better able to handle the ups and downs of daily life.

> **Get REAL Note:** Never wait until that "special" time in the future to start feeling happiness. Decide to make the most of each moment you have. Part of the experience comes from the trip. So allow yourself to have fun. "Laughter doeth good like a medicine" is more than a proverb—it is a fundamental truth. Laughter releases pleasurable endorphins in the brain and boosts the immune system.

How long has it been since you really laughed? I mean the kind of laughter that makes you tear up or double over. Most adults have forgotten to make laughter and humor part of each day. That should be a tangible goal for every person. Studies show that happy, humorous people live longer and have less illness. So don't take yourself too seriously, even if the task at hand is serious.

Accept yourself just as you are now, even though there are improvements to be made. (There will always be things you want to improve.) Accepting where you are, on the way to where you are going, is a vital part of renewed thinking. Joyce Meyer says, "I'm not where I need to be, but thank God I am not where I used to be." You too can embrace this positive approach. Start by doing what you can do now. Give yourself permission to be where you are, and to like who you are or choose to do something about it! Those are the only two choices to achieve peace, if you seek balance in mind, body, and spirit.

> **Get REAL Point:** To succeed, you must change as the seasons of your life change.

Regularly evaluate your current situation, and seek the clarity to make informed choices. Be able to laugh, smile, and say "Oh well" when life hands you lemons. Being grumpy and sad always makes things worse. Be the kind of person you enjoy being around, and strive to give people more than they require of you. If that is not your normal personality, it may take some effort before this becomes a natural way of behaving.

One of the most overlooked areas of health improvement is the building of meaningful interpersonal relationships. Today's society values productivity and personal fulfillment. Lost is a sense of community and interconnectedness. There is great value in acknowledging people and asking them questions about themselves and their lives, then really listening and taking in what they tell you.

By investing in others, you can take your mind off yourself and your own frustrations. This can be extremely restorative. You don't have to wait to be asked—look around and see where you can help, encourage, and validate others. This shift in thinking will prove to set the tone for your healthier lifestyle.

Too often people become obsessed with the busyness of their own lives. They no longer make time to casually meet with others and build real relationships because they are too stressed or too "busy." Remember, you create your schedule. If you do not have time to sit with a neighbor for thirty minutes, relax, and have nice conversation—there is a problem.

It is through the building of this network of strong relationships that people find support and genuine fulfillment. Acquiring "stuff" or running to multiple practices and appointments are makings of busyness. Be careful to examine what you allow to fill your time and see if those activities align with your personal goals and what matters most to you. If they do not, you need to prune them.

When life is ruled by the "have-tos," there can be little enjoyment or room for real change. Lifetime wellness and a sense of well-being come from a change in thinking. If you have never been able to stick to a "diet" or make those REAL lifestyle changes, it is time to either decide to make it work this time or decide that you are okay with where you are now.

Fully realize what the alternative to healthy choices will bring you. Embrace your own accountability and responsibility! It is all about choice—choices only you can make. Consider that you will eventually harvest the bounty of whatever seeds you plant now. So plant wisely and use your time fruitfully to reap rewards in abundance.

> **Get REAL Note:** Sometimes when you feel "buried" in life, when things just seem like too much, you are really just being "planted." Consider this is a chance to grow. Keep your chin up, keep attending to your daily tasks, and you will reap the harvest.

My goal is to help people through education and motivation. I have been there, and I am often one of the worst offenders of all the concepts I teach. Even though I know what to do and why to do it, I don't always choose to! That is one of the reasons I speak so candidly. I have learned that accepting where I am at the time is a main factor in achieving a sense of well-being. If you always feel bad about yourself because you are not doing those healthy habits that you know you should do, but don't feel like doing, you will live in misery.

When it comes to losing weight, everyone does it differently. Take a group of people who all have the same goal, and their results will be diverse. Some people seem to be superachievers; they appear to lose weight effortlessly. Others will be hanging in there making steady, slow progress (these people tend to have the best long-term success rates). Some people will start strong and gradually slow in progress, while still others will fail to really get anything going.

You probably know where you fit in. Often you will get out of your efforts what you put into them. That said, remember this is a lifetime wellness marathon, not just a sprint to a size. Each person will set individual goals and will have different reasons for doing so. You are where you are for a reason. Some factors you can control and many you can't.

The ones who really struggle tend to glare at those who make huge strides. Why is that? It is because it does not seem fair. Does this mean the ones who are successful work harder or make more sacrifices? Absolutely not! Yes, those who lose weight easily or who always seem fit may work hard, but often the groups that don't see such dramatic results push even harder. Be sure to pay close attention to your personality traits that can help and hinder your progress.

> **Get REAL Note:** It is not a fair comparison to equate actual weight loss with actual work done or amount of sacrifice. It is comparing apples to oranges. So do not feel like you are doing a bad job because you do not match up with the results of someone else. You must evaluate your progress based on the goals you set and what you are individually capable of.

So why is there such a difference in results? It has to do with many factors and unknown variables. Some are:

- The amount of lean muscle you have.
- Your metabolic rate or metabolism (the rate at which you burn calories).
- Your family history (the genes you got).
- Any underlying health problems.
- Genetic conditions.
- Your prior manipulation of food intake.
- Your activity level (one of the most overlooked factors).

It is time to consider that maybe your high school weight is not a realistic target anymore. How many years has it been since you were at your "ideal" weight, and how have you maintained your physical health since then? You did not get the way you are now overnight. It took years of practicing poor habits. Assuming that a few weeks of better habits will fix what it took years to achieve is not realistic, if you think about it.

If you have always been pretty fit and healthy, but have recently let yourself go somewhat with some undisciplined eating and a reduction in your activity level, you might be a candidate for a speedy tune-up. You can return to your past condition if you begin making more disciplined choices and picking up your activity level. Your body will have deconditioned some, but it will still have a recent "memory" of your past fitness level and will more readily snap back to that condition.

But if you are like most folks and it's been a long time, if ever, since you made disciplined food and activity choices it will take a little longer for your body to adapt to your new lifestyle and start to transform into that image you have in your mind. Take that into account when looking at how others progress. All that said, remember to put your blinders on and do your own thing. You are a unique individual!

Get REAL Point: You must learn how to build a bridge to reach your goals.

Creating a healthy lifestyle is a lifelong journey. Most chronic dieters share a common thought process. They understand that they need to lose weight, and they would like to, but on some level they are comfortable with their bodies. Enjoyment of personal habits and the pleasure gained from the weight-causing behaviors keep them in bondage. To them, it is often more comfortable living life at that level than going through the struggles and hard work of trying to shed the weight and become more fit—not to mention the guilt and shame that can result if goals are not met.

It is tough to tell someone facing multiple stressors to give up the few habits that they are using to cope and deal with their stress. Taking that behavior away, while at the same time offering only a painful replacement, will never work. Until something more beneficial is found to replace the harmful behavior, people will want to lean on the familiar. If you are in that situation, you have two choices. You can remain where you are, a place of relative comfort, or you can aspire toward your goal. The problem is, there is no *easy* bridge from your comfort zone to your ultimate goal.

Get REAL Note:	For change to last, you must determine whether it is worth the hard work to reach your goal, or whether you are comfortable enough with where you are right now.

Many people start out on this journey and find it hard to navigate. So they return to the comfort and familiarity of their original situation. Giving up on the journey happens for many reasons. Most people who attempt this journey have not been equipped to deal with the obstacles that they will encounter. Knowing what to expect and having a plan to counteract problems will go a long way in propelling you toward a goal destination. You can then properly equip yourself to withstand the journey.

Being well equipped is an important part of building a bridge to your goals. In order to be successful, you must possess and use your tools to navigate the pitfalls of the trip. Build your bridge by using your knowledge of food, its effect on your body, how to exercise, and why it is important, along with the mental component of making healthy changes, to create a strong foundation. Use that bridge to access your goal destination in a way that allows you to enjoy and maintain your residence there.

> **Get REAL Tip:** Support your bridge with strategies and tactics that allow you to make wrong steps without falling completely off the wagon. (Who made "the wagon" such a good place to be anyway?)

After starting this journey several times, many people decide that it is easier to just stay at their current comfort level, at a less than ideal size, than it is to go through a period of uncomfortable change. Making the effort can become too much to deal with in their current situation.

At this time, the prize is not worth the cost of the journey. For this season of life, the journey is not a top priority. This struggle is especially true for women. They deal with multiple responsibilities and face issues that cause the release of hormonal and chemical reactions in the body.

Because all people are hardwired differently, each is affected differently by these reactions. If you struggle with food issues and your neighbor does not, it is safe to say you're not getting the same chemical or hormonal signals. These reactions, combined with multiple unforeseen variables, lead to a more complicated equation.

Learning how the body makes and responds to chemical cues is helpful information to have. Some of the chemicals that act in the body are defined in the glossary toward the end of this book. When you understand what is happening, you can develop a plan to battle these chemical invasions. Now is the time to discover ways of dealing with the specific pitfalls unique to your system.

It is amazing how much discomfort we will put up with when we are building something great. So it is with building the bridge to your goals.

Picture that healthier you, just as you would picture your new or remodeled home. Start with small actions that lead to big changes.

You need to realize what you have control over and what you don't. Use what you can control to offset what you cannot. By building a bridge of smart food choices, exercise discipline, personal relaxation and de-stressing, and working smarter, not harder, you can meet goals without being worn down on the journey.

People often falsely assume they must be motivated first and then act later, but often the motivation will come after the action. When you make small, doable changes and succeed, you will be motivated to do more.

Your trip across the bridge can be more comfortable when you utilize the tools you have learned about. Those tools will be unique to who you are. Use them to help you deal with the uncomfortable feelings associated with changes in lifestyle.

The journey to your goal may feel like a climb, but it shouldn't feel steep. You have an edge—you are equipped. You possess the tools you need to get where you want to go. You are on the right track; by reading this guide, you show that you are sincere in your efforts and desire to start on a personal journey.

Just what that journey is will depend on you. So get started—*now* is the time. Evaluate, plan, execute, and build a bridge that will result in the fulfillment of your total health goals. As my son would say, "Build a bridge, and get over it!"

> **Get REAL Note:** If your goal is serious weight loss and you want to see REAL results, you will have to work harder than people who only want to improve their health and fitness levels.

Often, frustration with previous attempts to change makes people skeptical of starting again. For some reason, their past efforts have failed. This is why it is important to know your goal. Slow and steady "Turtle Power" will improve your health and fitness over time. It is not a "lose weight quick—get healthy fast" concept.

This section is for those people who are ready for more, but think nothing will work for them. Often people say they are "really serious" about losing weight, but they aren't taking the best path to get where they want to be. If this is you, ask yourself these questions:

- What is my goal? In what time frame? Is this realistic?
- How bad do I want to reach this goal? Is the payoff enough?
- Am I willing to be uncomfortable to reach to this goal?
- Am I willing to make time for the changes that must be made?
- Can I handle changing my routine and lifestyle?
- Am I prepared to maintain any lifestyle changes?

If you answer no to any of the above questions, then making sweeping lifestyle changes to bring dramatic weight loss (a goal that many set) may not be your best approach. I often hear "I am disappointed. I have been really trying, but I am just not seeing the results."

I understand where you are coming from. You are restricting your food choices and sacrificing some of your favorite snack foods, and at this time, what you are giving up does not seem worth the minimal success you have seen. But so far, if your effort has only included restriction and sacrifice, you are likely to be disappointed with the results.

Get REAL Point:	The key issues discussed below are not meant to go against the moderation theory, but are listed to provide a "reality check" and define realistic expectations.

After talking to a diverse population of people, I have found a few basic key issues they have in common. Keep in mind that these are generalizations, but they apply to many people stuck in this situation. Here are some of the key issues that stall the progress of "yo-yo diet and weight-cycling" folks.

The vast majority are not exercising enough, if at all.

You can only decrease calories so much. (Eating too few calories actually stalls your metabolism, causing your body to adapt to the caloric decrease.) Your other alternative is to increase the number of calories you burn. Very few people are successful at losing weight *and* keeping it off without exercising almost daily! If you are having trouble losing weight, twenty minutes of exercise three times a week may not be enough. (It is great for your health and for maintenance, but not enough to produce continued weight loss.)

Making exercise a daily priority in your life increases your chances of continued weight loss and maintenance. Often those who have dramatic weight loss (excluding surgery and other weight-loss aids) are exercising an hour or more per day. They might split it up and do some exercise in the morning and some in the late afternoon or evening. Also consider the intensity of your efforts and aim to work in your target heart rate range.

You may need to "up" the intensity or change your activities if your body has adapted to what you do regularly. If you're having difficulty losing weight, try to average at least thirty minutes of exercise every day, ideally more, at target intensity until you reach your goal. You can build up to this, but realize what it will take to get there. If you want big results, you will have to put in big effort!

Most who are exercising are not weight training.

Weight training is critical to maintaining your muscle mass and tone. If you're not weight training while trying to lose weight, you will lose muscle mass and tone and your basal metabolic rate will decrease, causing you to burn fewer calories twenty-four hours a day! The multiple health benefits of weight training are well known. Incorporating it into your regular routine is a commitment you need to include in your plan.

Make it fun—break it into manageable pieces. Learn from someone who will properly instruct you. Proper form and use of the proper weight is imperative for seeing results from your work. Twice a week for forty-five minutes to an hour is enough for two total-body workouts. This can be broken up into four days at fifteen to thirty minutes a session. Even more versatile is a daily minimal routine done in short bursts of time throughout the day. This will need to be well structured and designed to target a total-body workout.

Pre-exhausting the larger muscles before focusing on the smaller groups will allow the smaller groups to work independently. This principle should be considered in any plan you choose. Varying the routine will prevent adaptation and keep your body challenged.

Many actually consume more calories per day than they think.

Some dieters exceed their calorie budget by over 500 calories per day! If you're not sure, write down *everything* you eat and drink for a few days. This is a good time for you to get reacquainted with portions, calorie counts, and food labels. Pay close attention to these things until you are more comfortable with what a portion is and the general calorie content of basic foods. Keeping an intake log and paying attention to what you are eating for a short time helps you note where your biggest weaknesses are so that you can address them. It is a Get REAL reality check! Don't forget to count the liquid calories and toppings. It all adds up and could be the cause of your weight creeping up.

Some actually consume more fat than they think.

Limiting *non-healthy* fat intake is important for everyone. Look for cooking methods to help you cut extra fat out of ordinary meals. Be mindful of the types of fat you consume, and try to avoid more than one high-fat splurge item in one day. Spread out your treats and enjoy them. Fat is calorie dense, and most kinds are nutritionally poor. Consuming large amounts of fat will greatly reduce the number of calories you will have left to spend on more nutritious items. Be moderate and balanced. Planning, not restricting, is the goal!

Most want instant results.

When instant results don't happen, many people either give up or go on some crazy diet. You have to be resolved to the fact that weight loss *will* be slow! You need to embrace "Turtle Power" to meet your long-term objectives and maintain them. Don't waste time on gimmicks. Use your time to set realistic expectations, set your mind and push yourself. Accepting this principle is like having a huge weight lifted off your shoulders.

Many often skip meals.

Skipping meals is bad because it slows your metabolism, causing you to burn fewer calories twenty-four hours a day. Try to take in food within the first ninety minutes of waking up. This will prevent the body from releasing those "starvation hormones" that cause the conservation of body fat. When the body sends chemical signals that it is very hungry, we often eat faster and eat more food to satisfy this intense need.

For best results, don't let more than three to four hours go by during the day without eating. Choosing a protein source or complex carbohydrate for breakfast will help maintain blood sugar and avoid that mid-morning crash. Aim for at least 100 to 300 calories in your morning meal. Adding calories now can reduce calories later. This will help keep those chemical signals in check.

Most consume far too many refined carbohydrates.

Refined carbohydrates include foods such as white rice, white (non–whole wheat) flour products, white (non–whole wheat) pastas, soft drinks, sweetened drinks, and the hundreds of products that contain added sugars, which can appear on ingredients lists with names like sucrose and high fructose corn syrup. These foods give you very few nutrients for the calorie content and are rapidly absorbed by the body. This rapid absorption spikes your blood sugar, which can cause a rebound crash.

These types of carbohydrates can leave you feeling hungry and craving more, a vicious cycle that leads to chronic overeating. To balance hunger and cravings, consider when and with what you consume sugars and other refined carbs.

Many consume far too few fruits and vegetables.

Neglecting this part of your diet causes a lack of vital nutrients. Your body metabolizes the vitamins that you get from food better than those from supplements. Our bodies are designed to utilize all the food groups for optimum performance. Fruits and vegetables provide needed dietary fiber and fill you up naturally. Learning to incorporate them into your daily diet is essential to any successful plan. Planning their consumption is part of building healthy habits. Look for simple ways to add fruits and vegetables to current choices. They are power fuel for the body.

Some don't want to give up or limit alcohol.

Alcohol is a triple whammy—it stimulates your appetite, slows your metabolism, and is loaded with calories! Alcohol also lowers your inhibitions, a situation that can lead you to make poor choices.

Many consume large amounts of highly processed foods or foods containing artificial additives and preservatives.

Additives and preservatives are found in most boxed or canned items. Nonperishable foods are able to stay on the shelf without spoiling due to preservatives that keep them stable. Look for and avoid partially hydrogenated oil and products that are bleached or enriched. The body doesn't recognize these altered substances readily, and as a result you may not get the fullness signal sent to your brain. When you balance your diet with natural foods, your body will respond more quickly to its natural hunger cues. Eating natural, whole foods regularly allows you to recognize those cues.

Most consume too many artificial sweeteners.

Artificial sweeteners stimulate the pancreas to release insulin, just like sugar would. Insulin causes your body to store fat and prohibits your body from burning fat for fuel. Yet because artificial sweeteners are low in calories, they do not give your body the same sense of fullness it receives from real sugar. This can lead you to feel hungry again soon. When you do not feel fullness, your chances of overeating are increased. These calorie savers can cause you to be a calorie craver later in the day!

Many always eat until they're full.

Aim to stop eating just before you're full, and see how you feel thirty minutes later. Chances are good that you will feel satisfied by that time. Purposefully not eating every bite on your plate is a good place to start.

Be sure to drink water to cleanse the palate. Brushing your teeth or chewing sugarless gum after meals can also reduce your urge to keep eating. Ditch the thinking, "If I don't eat it now, I might be hungry later." That type of thinking leads to overeating routinely. If you are hungry later, you can have a healthy planned snack. Remember, this is not about deprivation—you need to eat!

Many don't address being carb sensitive.

People who are carbohydrate sensitive (CS) need to eat in a way that reduces cravings and creates feelings of fullness. If this is not done, the CS person will always struggle with excess weight. Weight control will feel like a never-ending battle for the person sensitive to carbs who does not manage this condition. CS can be managed, but it requires learning about new ways of eating and being intentional in your choices. When you take the time to make plan-focused choices, you will see real results.

> **Get REAL Point:** Significant weight loss and eventual mainten-
> ance is difficult. A wise man once said, "A man
> will make time for what a man wants to make
> time for." And he was right! If weight loss is
> something you really want, you will make time
> for it in your lifestyle.

Most have hit and miss efforts and lack consistent commitment.

Let's face it, it easier to eat what you feel like eating when you have time to eat it. But in order to feel good, have energy, and be healthy, you will need to plan and prepare. That is where commitment to your Personal Wellness Plan comes in. It is important to grasp that you can achieve your goals slowly through the moderate, gradual, and consistent changes I have discussed. But if you want faster or more significant results, you will have to work harder.

It is important to be realistic when deciding what you to choose to do. I firmly believe that choosing to do what you can do, and building on that, is far better than burning out and doing nothing at all. If you are not ready to embrace this kind of thinking, then learn to embrace who you are—just as you are! Accepting who you are is an important step in moving forward and enjoying everyday life.

Many people try too hard to reach an unrealistic goal.

Often, people meet those elusive goals only when they stop trying so hard to reach them. It is important to have fun on the journey toward your goals. I hear people say "I just can't lose weight" all the time. To that I say, "You just have not unlocked a lifestyle that will support the change your body will respond to." But if you really want to change, there is a way.

The blueprint has been mapped out for you. It is now time to follow the plan you create. Beware—knowledge without action is dangerous. It leads to complacency. Instead of being spurred to act when reminded of the information again, you tend to gloss over it. For success, you need to *act* on the plan you have mapped out for yourself. Your flexible plan will become intertwined into a lifelong wellness lifestyle. Remember, it is your daily *lifestyle* that will ultimately determine the results of all your efforts. Shape your lifestyle to reshape yourself. Press through, stay accountable, and your potential is limitless.

> **Get REAL Bottom Line:** Know your goal, and realize that without an investment there is no return!

My mission is to *empower you* to make good choices for yourself. You are in control—and by accepting that, you can begin to have a fresh outlook on your situation. The old adage "If you teach a man to fish, he will never go hungry" has always appealed to me. If the only way you could stay healthy and fit was to have someone making decisions for you, it would be a limiting situation. But if I can teach you how to make better wellness-related decisions for yourself, then you can use that information to make REAL improvements in your daily life. This will allow you to be healthy and fit, in whatever situation you find yourself in.

I hope this guide has given you the resources and motivation to make creating a Personal Wellness Plan an enjoyable and rewarding experience, one that brings about REAL lifestyle changes that will last. Coming to terms with the reality of what you really want is part of the process. You hold the key to unlock your goals—it is up to you to decide whether or not you will turn it.

GET REAL SUMMARY

This entire book has focused on a philosophy, a "Get REAL" approach to traditional health and wellness teaching. The following is a summary of the heart of this philosophy and the founding principles that were used to construct the contents—the "at a glance" version of what I believe. This information should summarize the basis for many of the concepts offered, along with refreshing some key points. My best to you on your personal journey toward lifelong wellness! It is all in you, just waiting to emerge.

 Traditional weight-loss diets do not work.

Well, diets may work temporarily, but not in the long term. Why? Because no one will continue to live in deprivation and restriction. As you return to "normal living," you will eventually gain back what was lost, plus some.

Why plus some? Because weight that is lost quickly is not all fat. Muscle is lost as well. The body is not capable of dumping that much pure fat in such a short time. As the previously lost weight is regained, the metabolism will now be less efficient due to the reduced muscle mass (because muscle helps burn calories at a faster rate). Long-term dieters educate their fat cells to store fat. They are now worse off than before trying to lose weight. The suffering will be for a temporary gain and can cause long-term frustration. This leads to yo-yo cycling of weight, which severely damages the body's metabolism and response to hunger.

Keeping your metabolism revved up, not stalled out, is essential to maintaining a healthy long-term relationship with food.

Studies show that your metabolism increases as you eat more and gain weight, and it decreases as you eat less and lose weight. In an attempt to maintain homeostasis, your body will adapt to the number of calories that you regularly consume. If you stay on a long-term restriction plan, you may get stuck there. Any deviation will cause the dreaded weight gain.

The only way to bust out of this sad situation is to go ahead and eat. You will gain some weight at first. However, by combining an increased healthy calorie intake with regular exercise, you will begin the process of resetting the damage you have done through past overrestriction. During this time, you can add *short* periods (up to seventy-two hours) of reduced-calorie eating.

A diet? Maybe, but think of it more as a tool to stave off "starvation hormones." By weighing weekly and utilizing a three-day calorie reduction to take off the extra pounds that show up, you will keep your metabolism on track for the long haul.

 The battle of the bulge is often a battle of the *mind* more than the body.

If you are not in the frame of mind to make small, consistent lifestyle changes, you will not find the success you desire in the long run. Life is what you make it. You need to have the energy to enjoy every day of it. Grumpy, dieting people are *not* fun to be around. They constantly talk about what they can't have, want to have, and need to do. This behavior keeps the brain on food and sacrifice!

Remember that what you keep your mind on is what you will attract to yourself. Always focus on the good you are *adding*, not that which you are limiting. When you spend time adding the good things, the negative things become less important. Think about what you are thinking about. It is time to get off the judgment wheel.

Constant negative self-talk (internal dialogue) leads to feelings of failure for not living up to the way you think you "should" live. Remember, don't "should" on yourself! Always thinking about how you "should" do this or "should" do that leads to constant frustration and prevents progress. Learn to forgive missteps and make corrections at the next opportunity. Improving wellness is a mental and physical experience.

 For results to last, you must determine what consistent changes you are willing to stick to—day in and day out.

You must change your mindset from restriction and deprivation to small, daily modifications. Decide what is actually doable for you. Just because someone tells you "this is the standard" does not mean that is where you must start. Health and wellness are by-products of small endeavors repeated consistently, day in and day out. See what just a few small changes, done consistently for a length of time, will yield.

For example, by consistently taking in fifty fewer calories daily or burning an extra fifty calories per day, you can lose five pounds in a year. The opposite is also true. If you take in an extra fifty calories per day, you will gain those five pounds in a year. Yikes! You can see how consistently changing your habits even just a little will affect your waistline.

Set REAL goals, even if they are below what fitness books or experts tell you.

If you wait to start your weight loss program until you have more time to commit to it, you will never do it. Do what you can and will do now, and then add to it later if you choose. Too much too fast always sets you up to crash! This is the missing link in most failed plans. There is such value in increasing aerobic endurance, building lean muscle, and improving your nutrition!

Now is the time to set those REAL goals and begin. How do you eat an elephant? One bite at a time. Don't be overwhelmed by the big picture. Just bite into it and keep chewing! Eventually you *will* meet your goal, *if* you do not give up. You have to start somewhere. No excuses—start today and stick with it!

 Learn the supreme value of moderation.

You will never succeed with an all-or-nothing attitude, because you are either absorbed in your plan or you have chucked it. Either way, you are setting yourself up for failure. Life is a marathon, not a sprint. Remember the story of the tortoise and the hare, and embrace your inner "Turtle Power!"

Almost everyone gets "hare syndrome" when it comes to healthy living attempts. We start out at full speed, but get so worn out from the all-out effort that we end up taking a little nap along the way. Remember, in the end, the turtle wins the race. Allow your efforts to be more turtle-like, slow and steady. Slow and steady wins the long-term race, after short-term leaders have fallen by the wayside.

Focus on fitness, not fatness.

Being fit and healthy is much more important than being thin or just looking good. I know many naturally thin people who are neither fit nor healthy. In the genetic lottery, they won a highly efficient metabolism. Down the road, however, this can turn out to be a problem for them. Since they do not have the outside social pressure to exercise, they often miss out on all the health benefits it can bring.

Just as there are unhealthy thin people, there are also very fit and healthy fuller-figured people. As the saying goes, "Don't judge a book by its cover." It's what's going on inside that matters. This is what will ultimately affect how you look, feel, and perform daily. Being able to walk up a flight of stairs, lift a child, or fight off an illness is a gift that money cannot buy.

When you eat right and exercise to improve your health and fitness, you will see the most REAL benefit for your time. The exterior will take care of itself. Get right on the inside, and you will be able to live a longer, stronger, and more joyful life.

 Food is your friend and your fuel.

Don't overly restrict your food options. Focus on the quantity and quality. Choose your food carefully and purposefully. Make eating whole, unprocessed and unenhanced, foods a regular part of your day. Learn to enjoy processed foods in moderation. People tend to think they must totally sacrifice true food wants, and then they end up giving in (eating too much) and feeling like a failure. There is a better option.

You must learn how to enjoy good-tasting food and feel good about it. Learning how to eat so that emotions do not cause pleasure-food seeking is difficult, but it can be done. Make it a priority to eat for health rather than taste, and you will develop your own healthy tastes. Plan your eating to ensure that your body's daily nutritional needs are met. This involves learning about how your body responds to certain foods and uncovering your food habits. Developing intentional eating will allow you to eat what your body needs and respond to natural cues.

 Don't be fooled by the pleasure response to food.

When foods are eaten that you enjoy, it creates a pleasure response in your brain that is comforting. When you eat the same kind of food again, it will trigger that "food = happy" association. This is a strong chemical reaction! When you are low on the feel-good brain hormones, you will get the urge to eat those comfort foods. This is the body's way to recreate that pleasurable feeling. Your mission is to create new programming that associates things other than food with comfort and pleasure.

 Learn about carbohydrate sensitivity and determine whether it is an issue for you.

How you eat and plan your diet will be greatly influenced by this information. Go through the section of this guide that talks about carbohydrate sensitivity and see if you fall into that category. If you are carbohydrate sensitive, you will want to gear your changes toward balancing the carbohydrate-insulin-serotonin connection. Learning about what causes your hunger and fullness cycle is important. Use this knowledge when choosing a healthy eating style that fits you.

Don't overly restrict calories.

I want to cry when I hear women say they eat only 1,000 calories a day and still can't lose any weight. Over time, this pattern can severely alter your metabolism. As your body adapts to this meager calorie intake, it will actually signal a need to store more fat. The body senses that you are starving, which you are, and it will hold on to every ounce of fat it has. What was meant to protect you during the "survival of the fittest" days is no longer beneficial during this time of plentiful food options. The body will work to protect your "set point," and this creates a "push-pull phenomenon" (see Glossary). If you are in this situation, you will require a serious lifestyle overhaul to reset your delicate metabolism.

 Embrace activity.

The changes that exercise brings to your body are incredibly beneficial to your overall health. Your challenge is to find activities that you will stick to and benefit from. Start associating exercise with *fun* activity and things you enjoy. Stop the exercise you associate with *work*. It is time to create positive movement memories! Look for fun and nontraditional ways to get moving. A moderate and enjoyable plan to improve your fitness level is essential.

Start to have fun with movement and experience "recess" again. Discover the incredible benefits that an improved cardiovascular system will bring. Building your endurance and stamina will add years to your life and life to your years! Begin to see the improvements by tracking your progress through timed distances and heart rate monitoring. You will be encouraged to set goals and meet them.

Get hooked on resistance training.

This guide will give you some basic "get started" exercise plans. If you need more, there are numerous books, magazines, and websites that will give you step-by-step workouts for any fitness level or situation.

Weight-bearing exercise is vital to overall health and can halt or reverse the body's aging process. If you do not know what to do or how to do it, seek out help from someone who does. The possibilities are endless! Building lean muscle improves your body's overall functioning in ways that not only will improve health and manage weight, but can also prolong life.

 Once you find an exercise plan that you feel comfortable following—get to it!

For resistance training, start out two times a week. Come on, you can do that. Even ten or twenty minutes will be better than doing nothing. Once you have mastered that level of exercise, you can add more minutes, more exercises, more weight, or more days.

For cardiovascular exercise, follow one of the three plans mentioned in this guide. All are designed to gradually build your endurance and stamina. You will choose a plan based on your current fitness level. Build your experience and confidence slowly, and stick to it. You might even like it. If you go zero to sixty, you will burn out and go back to what you used to do—nothing.

Start taking time for yourself.

This needs to be a *nonnegotiable* part of your schedule. It is vital that you allow yourself the time you need to stay charged up. If your batteries are dead, you will be no good to anyone. This includes not only those you care for, but *yourself* as well. Being more stress resistant will help turn off those fat-storage hormones that come from chronic stress exposure. To be a truly healthy person, keep your cup filled up and overflowing. When this happens, you are able to give from the overflow, which helps you maintain your health while you give to others.

 Accept responsibility for your current condition.

It is time to stop complaining and blaming. Personal accountability is essential for progress to be made. Excuses are just roadblocks that halt growth. When you understand the actual roots of your healthy living issues, you can begin to deal with them. Until that happens, you will be doomed to keep fighting the same battles each time that you attempt healthy change. Acceptance empowers you to move forward and overcome your perceived past mistakes. Those same mistakes will become lessons and allow you to press past your past and press into your divine future. Many great opportunities await when you accept personal accountability and are willing to seek them.

 Surround yourself with things and people that support your new lifestyle.

Avoid buying those grocery-store magazines that have gooey recipes, stick-skinny models, and stories of how to "Shed 20 lbs. in Just Two

Weeks!" Replace them with *Shape, Fitness, Prevention,* or *Men's Health.* Fill your brain with ideas that support your new endeavors. The stories of success from REAL people who did it the right way, and the exercises and healthy recipes, will *reinforce* your new lifestyle, not make you long for what you have decided to change.

Groups like First Place, Weight Watchers, and TOPS (Take Off Pounds Sensibly) are helpful because of the support, encouragement, and accountability they provide. They reinforce the lifestyle you are trying to create and provide like-minded people a place to fellowship. A wellness coach or similar professional can also provide that needed support and guidance. Having an active social network is healthy and supports long-term adherence. It also reinforces social habits and behaviors. This creates a strong connection between mind, body, and spirit.

 Don't get stuck in the ruts of life.

Often people fall into bad habits as a result of lack of planning or due to uncontrollable circumstances that put them into a "survival" mode. When you are in survival mode, you are not going to be receptive to new ideas or changes. You are simply struggling to keep your head above water.

The problem comes when the situation improves, but you still continue in a survival, "just exist" mentality. You live like you did when barely making it. Even though you could do more or better, the old habits have become so comfortable that you can't seem to break out of what has become familiar and routine.

It is time to bust out of it! You must constantly reassess your situation and change to flow with it. Seeking outside help may make it easier to transition into your new life situation.

Value your ability to reassess, evaluate, adjust, and execute a modified plan.

This will help you transition through the ups and downs of life. Being adaptable can affect the way you look, feel, and live. We all know people who still have a hairdo or wardrobe from the eighties. You would like to tell them that it's time to update to this decade. But many of us practice the same personal habits we had back then and think nothing of it. It's safe to say that most people's lives and responsibilities are not the same as they were ten or twenty years ago. So your habits need to be updated and reflect that.

 Go with the flow, but stay on course.

Your Personal Wellness Plan must bend as your life changes and as you experience different life events. This is the secret to long-term success. Life is not static, and your idea of wellness should not be either. If you have been out of shape for a while and have weight-cycled through a series of diets and other dramatic attempts to lose weight or become healthier, take heart. There is hope for you! Following the plan you create for yourself will help you fulfill your goals. Today is the day you "Get REAL" and change your total health and wellness!

APPENDIX A

Get REAL Nutrition Charts

Portion Equivalents for One Serving
Visual Reminders

- 3 ounces of meat=deck of cards or palm of hand
- 3 ounces of grilled or baked fish=checkbook
- 2 tablespoons of peanut butter=ping pong ball
- 1 ounce of cheese or meat=thumb
- 1 tablespoon=thumb tip
- 1 teaspoon=finger tip
- Medium apple=tennis ball, baseball or closed fist
- Medium fruit or ½ cup=a standard light bulb or ½ a baseball
- ½ cup of cooked grain, pasta, cereal or rice=½ a baseball
- 1 cup of ready to eat cereal=hockey puck or fist
- ¼ cup of raisins=large egg
- ½ cup of ice cream=tennis ball
- 1 teaspoon of butter=finger tip, 1 dice or a standard stamp
- 1-2 oz. pretzels (15 small twists, 7 regular)=cupped hand
- 1/3 cup of nuts=a loose pile in a medium take-out coffee lid
- 1 ounce of cheese=4 stacked dice
- 1 ounce of nuts=1 cupped hand full
- 1 pancake=compact disk
- 1 slice of bread=cassette tape
- 1 piece of cornbread=bar of soap
- 1 cup of mashed potatoes=closed fist
- 1 cup of salad greens=baseball

Caloric Needs Charts

This chart gives a general guide for:

- (ETCN) Estimated **total calorie** needs
- (EDCA) Estimated **discretionary calorie** allowance

Male/Female Age	Not physically active < 30 min. daily		Physically Active >30 min. daily	
Years old	ETCN	EDCA	ETCA	EDCA
Children 2-3	1000	165	1000-1400	165-170
Children 4-8	1200	170	1400-1800	170-195
Girls 9-13	1600	130	1600-2200	130-290
Boys 9-13	1800	195	1800-2600	195-410
Girls 14-18	1800	195	2000-2400	265-360
Boys 14-18	2200	290	2400-3200	360-650
Females 19-30	2000	265	2000-2400	265-360
Males 19-30	2400	360	2600-3000	410-510
Females 31-50	1800	195	2000-2200	265-290
Males 31-50	2200	290	2400-3000	360-510
Females 51+	1600	130	1800-2200	195-290
Males 51+	2000	265	2200-2800	290-425

Note: EDCA is part of ETCN—*Not* in addition to it.

Since physical activity increases calorie needs, those who are more physically active need more total calories and will have a larger discretionary calorie allowance (DCA).

From: www.mypyramid.gov

Get REAL Note: To lose one pound per week you must—reduce 500 calories per day

Foods That Enhance Total Wellness

Some whole and natural foods can actually promote better health. Our bodies were designed to utilize natural food sources for specific functioning. The body will readily recognize these foods and begin to use them for body functioning. Each food listed below has natural health enhancing properties and benefits. Adding any of them to your diet would be beneficial. For more specific information you can go to: www.mypyramid.gov

Whole wheat	Nuts, non-roasted
Garlic	Dairy, low-fat
Yogurt	Dark Chocolate
Butter	Cottage cheese
Pomegranate juice	Fish Baked/Boiled
Tomato sauce	Salmon
Brown rice	Spinach
Berries	Beans and Lentils
Oatmeal-not cut	Prunes
Lean cuts of meat	Egg whites
Cheyenne Pepper	Cinnamon
Green Tea	Water, non-carbonated
Red Wine	Vinegar
Tomato juice	Vegetable juice
Natural Honey	Lemon
Fruit—better fresh	Olive oil-better uncooked

Vegetables raw/steamed—better fresh (Choose a variety and those that are brightly colored or deep green)

> **Get REAL Tip:** Look at first five ingredients of any nutritional label to see the items *main* value.

Nutrition labels usually list the highest percentage ingredients first. When you see any of the above items you can feel good about the nutritional content. When you see any of ingredients on the next page, you may begin to question its relative nutritional value.

Common Problem Foods and Additives

Foods and additives are metabolized by the body in different ways. Ingesting some of these can cause people to not sense true fullness which can lead to overindulgence. Some foods or additives can also aggravate certain health conditions or do not promote health in general, when taken beyond moderation. Avoiding or greatly limiting foods containing the following is recommended.

- Partially hydrogenated oil
- Hydrogenated oil
- High fructose corn syrup
- Trans fat
- Saturated fat
- Sugars (often ending in ...ose)
- Salt/Sodium
- Artificial Sweeteners
- Margarine
- "Enriched" foods
- "Bleached" foods
- White Flour
- Caffeine
- Artificial colors and dyes
- Carbonation
- Phosphoric acid
- Preservatives/MSG

Get REAL Tip:	Take each day as a whole and try to avoid days that your diet is made up of too many substances from the problem list.

By balancing your consumption throughout the day you will feel better about your wellness efforts. By looking at **each day as a whole** you can choose foods to balance what was consumed at earlier eating episodes. Consider the ratio of problem foods and additives to foods that enhance total wellness in your daily diet. In general try to add more enhancers and limit or avoid the potential problem causers. Make your goal to fill in any nutritional gaps at other eating episodes. This is where planning can be very beneficial.

Get REAL Nutrition Tips

1. All foods in moderation.

2. Make small changes in your lifestyle, not huge changes in your diet. You must enjoy life and have the energy to live it.

3. Make your best food choices on routine days. Save the splurges for special occasions. It is not what we eat in one day that gets us in trouble; it is our pattern.

4. Determine if you are a "Grazer" able to eat small portions and snacks all day or an "Over Achiever" who once started eating continues eating until it is gone or you have eaten too much. This is important to know when planning successful routine days.

5. Eat the foods you like but watch the portions. If you think, "I know I should not eat this," then only eat a reduced amount or skip it. Especially if it is a known "trigger food" (always causes you to overeat) for you.

6. Watch out for foods that make you crave other foods or larger portions, usually highly processed foods or simple sugars eaten alone. Know yourself, your trigger foods and personal weak areas.

7. Cut food in half. Tell yourself if you still want it in 20 minutes after you are done eating, then you can have it. Chances are you won't.

8. Do not deprive yourself of food indulgences. Do it smart and remember to balance it over the day.

9. Drink water all day. Look for ways to make water taste better to you, but avoid caffeine. Caffeine dehydrates (takes water from) the body.

10. Drink a glass of water before and after your meal. It cleanses the palate and helps fill you up.

11. If you make poor food choices at one meal, make better ones at the next meal. Never "scrap" the day over a poor set of food choices. Each meal starts a new chance to make more "plan-focused" choices.

12. Cut up vegetables as soon as you get home from the store. This increases the likelihood you will choose them. Also that you use them before they spoil.

13. Keep carrots and celery CUT UP in the fridge. Put them in convenience size bags. Make it handy.

14. Chew sugar-free gum to fight off the urge to snack. Xylitol, found in some brands of gum, can actually help to clean and protect teeth.

15. Brush your teeth after eating. Removing the food taste can fight off cravings.

16. Buy a few good pieces of fruit (avoid jumbo bags) and keep them handy. Savoring the rich and fresh flavor will create a positive food memory.

17. Choose foods as close to their natural form as possible for maximum health benefits.

18. Try meal replacement bars for meals on the go or a more healthful way to have chocolate. Look for ones that balance protein with the fat and carbohydrates.

19. Don't eat junk food at home regularly. Save treats for times when you are not at home. Not having junk handy will decrease boredom eating.

20. Order the kid's meal. You could have three *Kids Meals* for the fat and calories in most super sized *Adult Meals*.

21. Make small changes in your shopping. Evaluate labels and buy "light" only occasionally. Avoid fat-free unless you just particularly like it, due to the additives they put in to make it more palatable.

22. Eat your largest meal early in the day when possible.

23. Make soda pop a treat and not part of the everyday routine. Carbonation is bloating and phosphoric acid is damaging to bones and teeth. It can often increase your hunger.

24. Ask for the "lunch portion." Many restaurants will do this if asked.

25. Watch eating too many processed foods. Look at the salt content, additives and preservatives. They can affect your appetite and overall health.

26. Make and order simple foods. The less complicated, without multiple ingredients and sauces, the better. You will feel fuller and reduce overeating.

27. Limit breaded and fried foods. When possible choose grilled, baked or broiled.

28. When enjoying fried foods, monitor the portions and keep the rest of the meal lighter in nature. Avoid multiple fried items at a time.

29. Never skip meals. You need fuel to function at your best. Your body runs best when it has balanced nutrition spread evenly throughout the day.

30. Eat off a smaller plate or bowl when possible. Visual trick. Good for members of the "clean plate club."

31. Use sugar and sweets sparingly. Try to pair them with a protein, dietary fat or complex carbohydrate. Try a glass of milk with that cookie. It is better to add them to a meal than to eat them alone.

32. Cut up your food into small pieces and savor each bite. Set your fork or sandwich down between bites. Taste the food and enjoy it.

33. Avoid eating a big meal three to four hours before going to bed. It does not metabolize as well and can decrease good sleep.

34. Stop thinking, "If I don't eat it all now, I'll be hungry later." This thought forces many to keep eating past actual fullness.

35. When faced with temptation, visualize the healthier looking you and see it clearly. Decide what you want more.

36. Split up large portions and eat the rest at another time. This is better digested than eating a large amount in one sitting.

37. Never eat a food you don't like (just because it is good for you) in place of one that you are craving.

38. Put up motivational things where you will see them such as the bathroom mirror, across from the toilet stool, kitchen, car dash, desk, locker, and etcetera.

39. If you eat when you get bored, find a diversion, any hobby or activity that will keep your mind and hands busy.

40. Know the calorie and nutrition contents of your favorite fast foods so you can weigh your options when eating out.

41. Eat slowly, eat slowly, eat slowly! If you must hurry, eat slowly and eat less. Your body needs time to digest what it takes in so that it can tell your brain it is full.

42. Practice leaving a few bites on your plate.

43. Enjoy conversation while eating. This promotes good digestion and a feeling of fullness. Social interaction has many benefits and naturally slows your pace.

44. Monitor your internal dialogue, that little voice in your head. When you see your meal, think to yourself, "I'll never be able to eat all of this!" Purposeful thinking versus, "This is so good I'll have to eat more," or "I'll start working on my eating next Monday." Changing your mental dialogue can influence behavior.

45. Avoid seconds. Eat only what you get on your plate the first time. It is more than enough. If you enjoy the food being served, make another small plate and put it in the fridge for a later meal or snack.

46. Note how many calories are in your favorite junk snack foods and compare that to how much exercise you would have to do to work it off. Decide if it is really worth it.

47. Have certain food combinations that are your "go-to meals," requiring you to make few decisions.

48. Reduce guilt over any perceived poor food choices. Always move forward and make better choices at the next opportunity.

49. Take time to evaluate what you want to gain from eating. Are you really hungry or is it boredom, unhappiness or low energy?

50. Take a daily multi-vitamin. Ensure adequate amounts of Vitamin C, Vitamin E, B Complex, and Folic Acid. Consider Vitamin C

that is esterized, Vitamin E with mixed tocopherols and a vitamin and mineral supplement that has been chelated. (Consult with your physician)

51. Take a daily mineral supplement Look for minerals as amino acid chelates. Important minerals to consider would be Calcium, Magnesium, Potassium, Zinc, Manganese, Chromium and Selenium. (Consult with your physician)

52. Look to add more fiber through complex carbohydrates and fruits and vegetables. Carefully evaluate the *first five* ingredients listed to ensure the actual "whole grain" content and to determine the bulk nutrients.

53. Think more *brown* and less *white.* Try whole grain options in your bread, crackers, pasta and flour. Choose brown rice over white and dense carbs over light and airy.

54. Add more nutritional value to common foods. Consider products such as protein powder, flax seed meal and wheat germ as non-flavor health additives to your recipes, cereal, yogurt, and smoothies.

55. Try adding pureed fruits and vegetables to regular recipes such as a cauliflower puree, blueberry puree and white bean puree. Even baby food can add a little extra nutrition.

56. Gear your mind toward *adding* more nutrition to each eating episode. Think of healthful additions to round out meals.

57. Remember, a meal is eating two or more *nutritious* foods at one sitting. At a minimum, it should consist of a complex carb and a protein. Having four or five different food options is *not necessary*

to constitute a meal. In fact, people tend to eat more, the more options they have, so keep it simple.

58. Try a baked potato *with the skin* before bed (3 hours after last meal). It helps the body raise your serotonin level. It creates an insulin response, which has an effect on the movement of the amino acid tryptophan from your blood into the brain. Choose any non-protein toppings and eat the skin.

59. Plan grocery shopping with the P2B ratio (7g protein to 15g carbohydrate) in mind. Create easy-to-grab snacks and take-along meals for easy access.

60. Have your "go-to" snack combinations either written down or thought up, for always ready snack ideas. Plan ahead—make it easier on yourself by pre-packing snacks ahead when you have time.

61. Make and split up several servings ahead of time and freeze them in individual serving sizes. This saves time in a crunch. Often those easy to grab, shelf-stable foods will trigger strong cravings.

62. Double healthy recipes and freeze them for when you are short on time.

63. Consider weekly meal planning. Write down meals that you plan ahead of time. It will help you to have needed ingredients on hand and increase your chances of sticking to your goals.

64. Take responsibility for what you put in your mouth. "Go ahead, eat *whatever* you want. It is your *butt*...ALL of it!" It is your body. You can do with it whatever you choose, for bigger or smaller.

65. Relish your freedom to choose and experience the enjoyment that comes from making wise choices within sensible boundaries. Be empowered by moderation and knowing that no food or food group is off-limits. Embrace the REAL control you have.

APPENDIX B

Get REAL Fitness Charts

Waist/Hip Ratio

Knowing where your body carries fat is important in understanding your risk of various diseases. People who carry their fat in the abdominal region (apple-shaped) have greater health risks than those who carry fat primarily in the hips and thighs (pear shaped). This type of visceral fat storage surrounds the vital organs and too much of it causes havoc in your body.

So what exactly is visceral fat? Your omentum is a fatty layer of tissue located inside the abdomen. It actually hangs *underneath* the stomach muscles and its main purpose is to store fat. Because the omentum lies underneath the muscles, this leads to the abdominal pooch or "pot belly."

It is soft and pliable because this fat is *inside* the body. The kind of fat storage we see in pear shapes is subcutaneous fat. It resides just underneath the skin's outer layer, thus making it less harmful to body functioning. When the omentum becomes so large and fatty it will actually start squishing and crowding the other internal organs out of the way.

> **Get REAL Point:** Your visceral fat is a good indicator of how you deal with chronic stress.

If you are under constant stress, your body releases high amounts of hormones into your bloodstream in the form of cortisol and adrenaline. Your body has to deal with these excess hormones, and this is your omentum's job. It takes these hormones from your bloodstream, and the hormones in turn step up the ability of your omentum to store fat. This results in a plump belly for you and internal disharmony.

The problem is that fat stored in this area is the first source of fuel for all of your internal organs, especially your liver. All of those added hormones throw off your metabolism by making you resistant to insulin, which means that sugar is floating around in your bloodstream instead of being used as normal by your cells.

This can result in tissue damage from chronically raised blood sugar. Your hormone balance is upset due to the abundance of inflammatory chemicals. This increased inflammation is due to fat being sent as a form of fuel directly to your liver, which in turn sends out the chemicals.

This creates inflammation throughout your system. It also causes "bad" cholesterol and triglyceride levels to rise by fueling your liver with its fat. So it is easy to see that having too much visceral fat is not only visually unappealing, but it is a serious health risk. Chances are if you have a rounded belly, or apple shaped body, your omentum is likely storing fat.

Machines that analyze body composition through bio-impedance are a way to measure visceral fat levels. It is not as accurate as a CT-scan but it is much more convenient and accessible. It can be a way to track personal changes. Another more convenient measure would be to determine your waist to hip ratio. You can use this as a guide to determine if you have increased risk for heart disease, hypertension and diabetes.

To calculate your waist/hip ratio (WHR): (in inches)

Divide your waist measurement by your hip measurement

- Men—Waist is measured at the navel
- Women—Waist is measured at the narrowest part of the torso—if not visible, use the navel

General classification of increased risk is defined as the following:

- Men=Waist to Hip Ratio WHR greater than 1.0
- Women=Waist to Hip Ratio WHR greater than 0.8

Indication of increased risk and need for weight loss, is a waist girth of:

- Females greater than 35 in. Males greater than 40 in.

Body Mass Index (BMI)

- Find your height in the left-hand column.
- Move across that row to your weight.
- The number at the top of the column is the BMI for that height and weight.

BMI	19	20	21	22	23	24	25	26	27	28	29	30	35	40
Height (in.)	*Find where height and weight meet to determine above BMI category.													
							Weight (lb.)							
58	91	96	100	105	110	115	119	124	129	134	138	143	167	191
59	94	99	104	109	114	119	124	128	133	138	143	148	173	198
60	97	102	107	112	118	123	128	133	138	143	148	153	179	204
61	100	106	111	116	122	127	132	137	143	148	153	158	185	211
62	104	109	115	120	126	131	136	142	147	153	158	164	191	218
63	107	113	118	124	130	135	141	146	152	158	163	169	197	225
64	110	116	122	128	134	140	145	151	157	163	169	174	204	232
65	114	120	126	132	138	144	150	156	162	168	174	180	210	240
66	118	124	130	136	142	148	155	161	167	173	179	186	216	247
67	121	127	134	140	146	153	159	166	172	178	185	191	223	255
68	125	131	138	144	151	158	164	171	177	184	190	197	230	262
69	128	135	142	149	155	162	169	176	182	189	196	203	236	270
70	132	139	146	153	160	167	174	181	188	195	202	207	243	278
71	136	143	150	157	165	172	179	186	193	200	208	215	250	286
72	140	147	154	162	169	177	184	191	199	206	213	221	258	294
73	144	151	159	166	174	182	189	197	204	212	219	227	265	302
74	148	155	163	171	179	186	194	202	210	218	225	233	272	311
75	152	160	168	176	184	192	200	208	216	224	232	240	279	319
76	156	164	172	180	189	197	205	213	221	230	238	246	287	328

(C.D.C. Calculations)

Get REAL Note: BMI can be inaccurate for those with large muscle mass or who are large boned. It does not account for the extra "healthy weight" caused by these factors. It should only be used as a tool and a reference.

Body Fat Percentage

Electrical Impedance devices are the easiest way for non-trained persons to determine body fat percentage. These can be purchased as a single device or are available in some scales. They work by estimating fat and muscle percentages from detected body water distribution.

Different tissues such as muscle and fat have different amounts of water, and therefore a different resistance to the weak current. Keep in mind this is not a fool-proof method. It provides a good way to track personal progress and can be a more useful measure than weight alone. It is not an accurate measure for person to person comparisons.

Skinfold Measurement

Skinfold Calipers provide an estimation of body fat using skinfold thickness measurements. It is easier to obtain than the final option which is **hydrostatic "underwater" weighing.** That technique is considered the "gold standard."

- When using calipers, only the right side is usually measured.
- Measurements are taken from **three to nine** different standard anatomical sites around the body.
- The tester pinches the skin at the appropriate site to raise a double layer of skin and the underlying adipose tissue, but not the muscle.

- The calipers are then applied 1 cm below and at right angles to the pinch, and another reading is taken two seconds later.
- The mean of two measurements should be taken. If the two measurements differ greatly, a third should then be done, then the median value taken.
- The reliability of skinfold measurement can vary by testers. It is best to use the sum of several sites to monitor and compare body fat measures.
- Skinfold calipers and a knowledgeable tester are required.

Goal Body Fat Percentage Formula

To determine the weight that meets your body fat percentage goal you can use this formula:

Goal weight= <u>Lean Body Mass</u>

                   1.00-Percent of Fat Desired

Example: A 160-lb. female has 25% body fat.

What should she weigh to achieve 15% body fat?

Fat weight=160 lbs x .25=40 lbs.

Lean Body Mass=160 lbs-40=120 lbs.

Goal Weight= <u>   120   </u> = <u>   120   </u> =**141 lbs.** would be 15% body
            1.00-0.15   0.85   fat for this person.

Risk of Associated Disease Waist Size and BMI

BMI	Risk Category	WHR </=40in. (men) </=35in. (women)	WHR >40in. (men) >35in. (women)
18.5 or less	Underweight	--	N/A
18.5-24.9	Normal	--	N/A
25.0-29.0	Overweight	Increased	High
30.0-34.9	Obese	High	Very High
35.0-39.9	Obese	Very High	Very High
40 or greater	Extreme Obese	Extreme High	Extreme High

- Note your BMI and determine your <u>Risk Category</u> based on that alone.
- Note your WHR across the top and your BMI down the side. Where the two lines intersect is you <u>Risk of Associated Disease</u> based on your WHR.

Sit and Reach Flexibility Test

This test measures the flexibility of the lower back and hamstrings. Lower back flexibility is important because tightness in this area is implicated in lumbar lordosis, forward pelvic tilt and lower back pain.

- This test involves sitting on the floor with legs out straight and shoes off.
- Feet are placed with the soles flat against a box, shoulder-width apart.
- A ruler or measuring tape is placed with the 0 at the feet level. The knees are held flat against the floor by the tester.
- With hands on top of each other and palms facing down, reach forward along the measuring line as far as possible.
- After three practice reaches, **the fourth reach is held for at least two seconds** while the distance is recorded. Ensure no jerky movements and that the fingertips remain level and legs flat.
- The distance reached by the hand will be scored to the nearest centimeter or half inch. This will depend on the scale being used.
- The reliability will depend on the amount of warm-up allowed, and whether the same procedures are followed each time.

Get REAL Note: Most variations of this test involve the differences in the value at the level of the feet.

The most logical measure is to use the level of the feet as recording zero, so that any measure that does not reach the toes is negative and any reach past the toes is positive.

- The **Presidents Challenge** procedures require that the box is made with 23 centimeters at the level of the feet, so 10 cm past the toes is recorded as 33 cm.

Sit and Reach Flexibility Chart

- This table gives you a guide for expected scores (in cm) for adults.
- It is using **zero** at the level of the feet.

Chart B-5:

	(Men)	(Women)
Super	>+27	>+30
Excellent	+17 to+27	+21 to+30
Good	+6 to +16	+11 to +20
Average	0 to +5	+1 to +10
Fair	-8 to -1	-7 to 0
Poor	-19 to -9	-14 to -8
Very Poor	<-20	<-15

Step Test

This test is designed to measure your **cardiovascular endurance.**

- Using a 12-inch high bench (or a similar sized stair in your house), step on and off for three minutes.
- Step up with one foot followed by the other, and then step down the same way.
- Try to maintain a steady four-beat cycle. It helps if you say "Up, up, down, down." Go at a steady and consistent pace.
- **At the end of three minutes,** remain standing while you immediately **take your pulse for one minute.** Use this ending heart rate (HR) to determine your cardio fitness level.
- Find your age across the top and your ending HR below that.
- Follow the line to the left to determine your cardio fitness level.

3 Minute Step Test (Men)

Age	(18-25)	(26-35)	(36-45)	(46-55)	(56-65)	(65+)
Excellent	<79	<81	<83	<87	<86	<88
Good	79-89	81-89	83-96	87-97	86-97	88-96
Above Ave.	90-99	90-99	97-103	98-105	98-103	97-103
Average	100-105	100-107	104-112	106-116	104-112	104-113
Below Ave.	106-116	108-117	113-119	117-122	113-120	114-120
Poor	117-128	118-128	120-130	123-132	121-129	121-130
Very Poor	<128	<128	<130	<132	<129	<130

3 Minute Step Test (Women)

Age	(18-25)	(26-35)	(36-45)	(46-55)	(56-65)	(65+)
Excellent	<85	<85	<90	<94	<95	<90
Good	85-98	88-99	90-102	94-104	95-104	90-102
AboveAve.	99-108	100-111	103-110	105-115	105-112	103-115
Average	109-117	112-119	111-118	116-120	113-118	116-122
BelowAve.	118-126	120-126	119-128	121-129	119-128	123-128
Poor	127-140	127-138	129-140	130-135	129-139	129-134
VeryPoor	<140	<138	<140	<135	<139	<134

APPENDIX C

Get REAL Cardiovascular Exercise Guide

Target Heart Rate Calculation

The most widely accepted mathematical formula to help you determine your target heart rate zone is known as the **Karvonen Formula.** This formula calculates a percentage of the heart-rate reserve, which is the difference between the resting heart-rate and the maximal heart-rate.

Get REAL Note:	This formula uses your maximum heart rate, multiplied by target percentages, to determine a target heart rate range. Staying within this range will help you work most effectively during your cardio workouts.

Calculating Heart Rate Reserve=(A-B=C)
(A) Maximal Heart Rate–(B) Resting Heart-Rate=(C) Heart-Rate Reserve

(A) **Maximal Heart Rate** is the highest rate a person should attain during exercise. For practical application an age-predicted heart-rate formula was developed.
MHR=(220–Age)

> **Get REAL Note:** This formula is based on the assumption that one's heart rate at birth is 220 and decreases by one every year. The accuracy of determining maximal heart-rate based on this formula can vary at any given age by plus or minus 10 beats per minute.

(B) Resting Heart Rate:

- Take your pulse for one full minute before getting out of bed in the morning or after resting for a few hours.
- Take this resting pulse for three to four mornings and average your results.

Determining Target Heart-Rates

(C) Heart Rate Reserve multiplied by the (% intensity) +(B) Resting Heart-Rate=**Target Heart-Rates**

Karvonen Formula Example:
36-year-old, resting heart rate of 65 beats per minute.

220-36 (Age)=184 (MHR)
184- (Resting Heart Rate) 65=119 (Heart Rate Reserve)

(65%) low end of heart rate zone = 119 x **65%**=77

77 + (Resting Heart Rate) 65=142
142 beats per minute would be working at 65% of your target heart zone.

(85%) high end of heart rate zone=119x**85%**=101

101+ (Resting Heart Rate) 65=166
166 beats per minute would be working at 85% of your target heart zone.

Target Heart Rate Zone for this person would be 142 to 166
For more information, see www.americanheart.org.

Target Heart Rate Zone using a Ten-Second Count

	(Example: Age-50 RHR-55)	
	220	220 Maximum Heart Rate Rule
-	40	Age
=	170	Maximum Heart Rate (MHR)
-	55	Resting Heart Rate (RHR)
=	115	Heart Rate Reserve (HRR)
x	60%	x Exercise Intensity
		(Sedentary 40-65% or 70-85%)
=	69	
+	65	Resting Heart Rate (RHR)
=	124	
÷	6	For the 60 seconds in a minute
=	20.66 or **21**	10 second count

Ten Second Heart Rate Chart

(As seen on next page)

- ✓ *Choose Neck or Wrist for pulse point*
- ✓ Check pulse for 10 Seconds
- ✓ Find your age range in the first column
- ✓ Locate your 10 second pulse along that row
- ✓ Determine target heart rate % from top row

237

Ten Second Heart Rate Chart

AGE	55%	60%	70%	80%	85%
15	19	21	24	27	29
20	18	20	23	27	28
25	18	19	23	26	28
30	17	19	22	25	27
35	17	19	21	25	26
40	17	18	20	24	26
45	16	18	20	23	25
50	16	17	19	23	24
55	15	17	19	22	23
60	15	16	18	21	22
65	14	16	18	21	21
70	14	15	18	20	21
75	13	15	17	19	21
80	13	14	16	19	20
85	12	14	16	18	19
90	11	13	15	17	18

For more information, see www.americanheart.org.

Get REAL Exertion and Tiredness Scale (G.R.E.A.T.S.)

I created an easy to remember **Get REAL Exertion and Tiredness Scale** (G.R.E.A.T.S.), based on a 1-10 system.

	G.R.E.A.T.S. Scale
Level 1:	Relaxing with no work or effort
Level 2:	Moving at an easy and very comfortable pace
Level 3:	More movement that produces increased breathing
Level 4:	Perspiration forming (Able to talk to someone without effort)
Level 5:	Increased perspiration, less comfortable (Able to talk easily)
Level 6:	Working harder (Slightly breathless)
Level 7:	Increased breathing, effort and fatigue (Able to talk but with effort)
Level 8:	Performing at an intense level (Heart rate, breathing and fatigue are high)
Level 9:	Heightened performance level (Can only be maintained for short period of time)
Level 10:	Maximum output and intensity level

> **Get REAL Note:** While doing physical activity, rate your "perception" of exertion. Choose the number that best describes your effort.

Note how difficult or strenuous the exercise feels to you, consider: physical stress, effort and general fatigue. Use the GREATS scale to reach your desired intensity range. It allows you to self-monitor and to alter your movements to meet your intensity goals.

For *most workouts,*
- You want to aim for a level **5 or 6.**

For *cyclical type exercise,*
- Your intensity peaks between **8 and 9**
- Your recovery period should be around a **4 or 5**

For *longer, slower workouts,*
- Your maximum perceived exertion (MPE) should be at level **5 or <5.**

> **Get REAL Note:** Working at a level 10 isn't recommended for most workouts.

Get REAL 10-Minute Cardio Blitz

In today's fast paced society many people forgo exercise because they don't feel they have enough time to devote to it. What they actually mean is, they don't think they could see any REAL results in such a short amount of time, so why bother? But that does not have to be the case. By varying the intensity of your workout you can see REAL results in just a short amount of time.

For this 10 Minute Blitz you will use the G.R.E.A.T.S. scale from the previous page. You will vary the intensity for each minute to provide a heart healthy workout. You will need a watch to keep track of the time. This can also be done using stairs.

*S.A.F.E. Stationary And Fast Exercise such as, jumping jacks, half jacks, step ups, running in place, and jumping in place.

Cardio Blitz	
Minute 1	Warm up/brisk walking G.R.E.A.T.S of 2-4
Minute 2	Fast walk with arm swing G.R.E.A.T.S of 5-7
Minute 3	Full running G.R.E.A.T.S of 7-8
Minute 4	(S.A.F.E.) of choice G.R.E.A.T.S of 7-8
Minute 5	Fast walk with arm swing G.R.E.A.T.S of 7-8
Minute 6	Full running G.R.E.A.T.S of 8-9
Minute 7	(S.A.F.E.) of choice G.R.E.A.T.S of 8-9
Minute 8	Full running G.R.E.A.T.S of 7-8
Minute 9	Fast walk with arm swing G.R.E.A.T.S of 5-7
Minute 10	Cool down/slow walk G.R.E.A.T.S of 2-4

Get REAL Cardio-Sculpt Track Workout

2 laps-walk

<u>Step ups</u> each leg-30 seconds (Use a bench or step, step up and down)

4 laps-walk

<u>Wall pushups</u> or bench pushups-one minute (Use a wall or bench)

1 lap jog

<u>Dips</u>-30 seconds (Use a bench or chair)

4 laps-walk

<u>Lunges</u> each leg-30 seconds (Use a step or flat ground)

1 lap jog

<u>Squats</u> or sit and taps-one minute (Use a bench or chair)

4 laps-walk

<u>Plies</u>-one minute (Stand behind a bench or chair)

2 laps walk

Stretch

Get REAL Note: You may adjust the lap count based on the size of the track.

Cardiovascular and Aerobic Activity Considerations

You should gradually increase your amount of cardio-time as endurance builds. Just because you can do more than suggested, does not mean that you should. It is important to go slow and not overdo it. You do not want to get burned out. It needs to become an enjoyable part of your lifestyle. That will not happen overnight, you must build it into your daily routine over time.

Get REAL Note:	On maintenance your goal should be at least 30 minutes, 4 times a week. Experts often recommend a minimum of 120 minutes per week for optimal health.

Be sure to *warm up* prior to starting your activity. You body temperature must be taken into consideration before beginning. Cold muscles will not cooperate as well as if they were previously warmed up. If you want to exercise in the morning, you can take a hot bath or shower as a passive way to raise your core temperature. It is not as efficient as doing five-plus minutes of light cardiovascular moves but it will elevate the muscle's temperature at the surface level.

You also need to add a *cool-down period* after you are done. The most efficient way of slowing down a car or bike isn't by riding straight into a brick wall. In the same way; you need to gradually slow down your body after a workout or exercise. Five to ten minutes of slow, easy activity will help your body recover from a workout. Your cool-down routine should include light cardio activity and stretching. Cooling down and stretching at the end of a workout help to:

- Slow your heart rate to a normal speed
- Return your breathing to its regular pace
- Avoid stiffness and soreness of the muscles
- Reduce any risk of dizziness and lightheadedness
- Relax the muscles

Whether you are new to working out or a long time exerciser, adding a good before-and-after routine will give you the best chance of avoiding injuries and may even help improve your performance. You can do cardio every day. Even if it is 5 minutes, it helps. It all goes toward your weekly total. You can also break it up in to multiple short sessions throughout the day. It still burns calories, fat and boosts the metabolism.

Get REAL Note: Your maximum benefit is achieved after 20 minutes of exercise. Work beyond that point is **enhanced fat burning**—making your metabolism go into overdrive. Keep that in mind when budgeting your time.

#1 Beginner Cardiovascular and Aerobic Activity

WEEK	Suggested Total Minutes	Possibilities
One	40 min	10 min/day-4 days
Two	50 min	10 min/day-5 days
Three	60 min	10 min/day-6 days
Four	80 min	20 min/day-4 days
Five	100 min	20 min/day-5 days
Six	120 min	30 min/day-4 days
(Can be achieved in 5 minutes increments)		

CARDIO/AEROBIC activity is any activity that will elevate your heart rate for a sustained time. This includes from your preferences: (* add your own ideas)

*Walking, brisk pace and using arms.　　　　*＿＿＿＿＿＿＿＿＿＿

*Stair climbing　　　　　　　　　　　　　　*＿＿＿＿＿＿＿＿＿＿

*Treadmill or exercise bike　　　　　　　　*＿＿＿＿＿＿＿＿＿＿

*Yard work (vigorous)　　　　　　　　　　*＿＿＿＿＿＿＿＿＿＿

*Trampoline jumping　　　　　　　　　　　*＿＿＿＿＿＿＿＿＿＿

*Dancing (continuous)　　　　　　　　　　*＿＿＿＿＿＿＿＿＿＿

Choose any combo of these or just one of these. You may combine if you do not allow too much time in the transition. (Heart rate must remain elevated) In the beginning of each week you should use your calendar to schedule cardio (in pencil) for that week. This will help you budget your time. Then use a pen to record when actual exercise was done.

245

#2 Moderate Cardiovascular and Aerobic Activity

WEEK	Suggested Total Minutes	Possibilities
One	80 min	20 min/day-4 days
Two	120 min	30 min/day-4 days
Three	160 min	40 min/day-4 days
Four	200 min	40 min/day-5 days
Five	225 min	45 min/day-5 days
Six	270 min	45 min/day-6 days

CARDIO/AEROBIC activity is any activity that will elevate your heart rate for a sustained time. This includes from your preferences: (* add your own ideas)

*Walking, brisk pace and using arms.   *_____

*Elliptical exercise machine, Treadmill etc.   *_____

*Swimming, sustained motion   *_____

*Exercise bike (stationary or outside)   *_____

*Aerobics tape or class   *_____

*Stair climbing   *_____

*Vigorous house or yard work (sustained) raking, vacuuming, etc.

Choose any combo of these or just one of these. You may combine if you do not allow too much time in the transition. (Heart rate must remain elevated) In the beginning of each week you should use your calendar to schedule cardio (in pencil) for that week. This will help you budget your time. Then use a pen to record when actual exercise was done.

246

#3 Weight Loss Cardiovascular and Aerobic Activity In Training (Conditioning Phase)

WEEK	Suggested Total Minutes	Possibilities
One	120 min	30 min/day for 4 days
Two	160 min	40 min/day for 4 days
Three	200 min	50 min/day for 4 days
Four	250 min	50 min/day for 5 days
Five	300 min	50 min/day for 6 days
Six	360 min	60 min/day for 6 days
Seven Plus	420 min	60 min/day for 7 days

CARDIO/AEROBIC activity is any activity that will elevate your heart rate for a sustained time. (Above is a training pace.) This includes from your preferences: (* add your own ideas)

*Walking/running, brisk pace and using arms. *_____

*Elliptical exercise machine, Treadmill etc.　*_____

*Swimming, sustained motion　　　　　　　*_____

*Exercise bike (stationary or outside)　　　*_____

*Aerobics tape or class　　　　　　　　　*_____

*Stair climbing　　　　　　　　　　　　*_____

Choose any combo of these or just one of these. You may combine if you do not allow too much time in the transition. (Heart rate must remain elevated) In the beginning of each week you should use your calendar to schedule cardio (in pencil) for that week. This will help you budget your time. Then use a pen to record when actual exercise was done.

Get REAL Stretching and Flexibility Considerations

Stretching can become a vital portion of your wellness routine. Warm-up stretches are necessary to prevent injury and prepare the body for more vigorous exercise. An active warm-up includes moving the large muscles of the body, mainly the arms, legs and back. A passive warm-up is accomplished by using hot baths, showers or saunas to raise the body temperature and warm the muscles. Some reasons to make stretching a part of your daily life include:

- Decreasing your risk of injury
- Enhancing joint mobility and integrity
- Increasing blood supply and nutrients to joints
- Better balance and coordination
- Improving situational awareness
- Deceasing risk of low back pain
- Improving range of motion and flexibility
- Preparing muscles for exercise
- Lengthening and relaxing muscles after exercise

Stretching exercises give you more freedom of movement to do the things you need and like to do. Stretching is important because it increases flexibility. This lessens the chance of injury and can also help you recover from injury.

Stretching allows the muscles to loosen, get prepared for the movement, and move with gentle ease through a wide range of motions as well as reduce the stiffness that can occur with exercise. It can also reduce stress and improve your feeling of wellbeing.

Stretching exercises alone can improve your flexibility, but they will not improve your endurance or strength. This makes stretching a valuable component of your overall fitness routine. It is essential to practice proper stretching techniques. Doing so will allow you to avoid any unnecessary injury. Tips to proper stretching technique include the following:

- Stretch prior to an exercise session. Do this only after you have warmed up for about five minutes. Stretching muscles when they are cold increases your risk of pulled muscles.
- Stretch after you do your regularly scheduled exercises. This helps to release muscle tension and lengthen the muscles.
- Do each stretching exercise one to three times.
- Slowly stretch into the desired position, as far as possible without pain. It takes time to lengthen tissues, so hold each stretch for 10 to 30 seconds—and up to 60 seconds for a really tight muscle or problem area.
- Never "bounce!" Instead, make slow, steady movements. Bouncing can cause muscles to tighten, possibly resulting in injury. It can cause small tears (micro-tears) in the muscle, which leave scar tissue as the muscle heals. The scar tissue tightens the muscle even further, making you even less flexible—and more prone to pain.
- Don't hold your breath while stretching. Relax and breathe deeply. Upon exhale you can deepen further into the stretch.
- Avoid "locking" your joints when you straighten them during stretches. You should always have a small amount of bend in your joints while stretching.
- Always warm up before stretching exercises (do a little easy walking or other gentle exercise). Warm muscles respond better to the stretch. Stretching your muscles before they are warmed up may result in injury.
- Establishing a set of morning and evening stretches can be very beneficial. They do not need to be lengthy or complicated to be of benefit. Simple stretches are equally effective.

- Stretching should never cause pain, especially joint pain. If it does, you are stretching too far, and you need to reduce the stretch so that it doesn't hurt. A mild pulling sensation is normal.
- Stretch both sides equally to make sure your joint range of motion is as equal as possible on each side of your body.
- If you have had a hip replacement, check with your surgeon before doing lower body exercises. Also, don't cross your legs or bend your hips past a 90-degree angle.

APPENDIX D

Get REAL Resistance Training Guide

Choosing the appropriate weight for each exercise is very important.

How Much Weight to Use?

➢ The amount of weight you use is dependent on the maximum amount of weight you can lift while keeping *proper form.*

➢ Your muscle should feel fatigued at the end of the sets, not strained.

➢ If your muscle is not fatigued (You could do many more reps without trouble), then you should *increase* the amount of weight.

➢ If you cannot make it to the end of the set using proper form, then you should *decrease* the amount of weight.

➢ Muscles should feel worked, but not *sore* or *over-tired.*

➢ You may need *different* weights for different exercises.

➢ It is better to do fewer reps with precision, than do many with flawed form (quality over quantity).

➢ Gradually increase the amount of weight used as you become tolerant (it is no longer challenging or producing results) of the current weight.

Common Training Definitions

DUMBBELL: Short bar with fixed weight on the ends

BARBELL: Long bar that can have weight added to the ends

REP: One repetition of the exercise (Beginning to end)

SET: Number of reps you do in succession (Usually 8 to 15)

MAX: Number of reps you can do in proper form

ISOLATION PAUSE: Done in the squeeze phase of the exercise. It causes focus on the area being worked

Get REAL Basic Training Tips

1. **It is best to start with lightweights of two to five pounds and then slowly progress the weight used as you train in the coming weeks.**

   - Gradual progression to heavier weights creates the sculpting of the muscles. Remember ladies, you won't "bulk up." It is not in your make up, you will only firm and define.

   - Exercise progression must be done slowly, steadily and consistently in order to effectively overload the muscles and reduce your chance for injury.

2. **To be most effective, an exercise routine should be steady and consistent.**

   - Sporadic exercising is common among many people. This will reduce the overall effect of the training.

- Starting out too gung-ho causes people to overdo it! The resulting soreness and possible injury will halt any future progress.

3. **For best results, have a plan to work specific muscle groups on certain days.**

   - Muscles need twenty-four hours to repair and rebuild. Note: this applies when fatiguing muscles and not just casually exercising.

   - Beyond twenty-four hours, your muscles begin to decondition.

   - Waiting too long to train again will reduce some of the benefit, depending on the amount of time that passes in between.

   - Training again too soon will not allow muscles to grow adequately. This can also cause overuse injuries.

Resistance Training Considerations

1. **Follow a "10 percent rule".** Don't increase the distance or duration of your workouts, or the amount of weight you lift by more than 10 percent each week. Use gradual progression.

2. **Always warm up.** It is important to warm up muscles prior to training in order to get the most out of your exercise and to prevent injury. Start your exercise sessions with at least 10 minutes of very easy cardio-exercise, such as walking or stationary cycling. Your muscles, tendons and ligaments can tolerate more stress when they are warm.

3. **Stretch each body part or parts after muscles have been worked.** To aid in stretching, elastic bands or a rolled up towel can be used.

4. **Start slow and allow your body to adjust to any new workouts.** Be sure to stretch and schedule recovery days to allow your muscle to heal and grow.

5. **Maintain proper posture.** Back straight with shoulders back, head high with neck relaxed and abdominal muscles tucked in. Think of a string that runs through you and out of your head and something keeps pulling up on it. Practice lifting your ribcage up out of your abdomen.

6. **Learn proper technique.** A trainer can teach you the subtleties of using exercise equipment, such as how to grip a weight bar, how low to squat and how to adjust a machine to fit your body. A couple of sessions with a trainer would be cheaper than a visit to an orthopedic surgeon. Small adjustments can make a big difference in the success of your workout program. If you still feel unsure about your technique, you can use weight machines rather

than free weights. They require less coordination than dumbbells, so they're safer for beginners.

7. **Avoid speed lifting.** Way too many people lift weights too rapidly. That is not very effective, because you're using momentum, not your own muscle power. Take at least two full seconds to lift a weight and two to return it to the starting position. Resist in both directions.

8. **Mix up your workouts.** People tend to go wild over one activity like weightlifting or cardio. Often doing the same things the same way will lead to the body adapting to it. This will not promote the most efficient training for your body. By varying your workouts, you will continue to challenge your body.

9. **Start by lifting lightweights.** Check your ego at the door. If you go too heavy, you'll have trouble walking the next morning. So choose a weight that fatigues your muscles after 10 to 12 repetitions. After a few weeks, you can graduate to heavier weights and drop down to eight to 10 reps—a range that ultimately will give you more strength.

10. **Listen to your body.** Know the difference between the slight muscle soreness of a good workout and the soreness that's a warning sign to get checked for injury. Good pain is achy, dull and very general. Bad pain tends to be sharp and specific.

11. **Rest!** People think that more exercise means more results, but when you over train, your body breaks down. Organize your weight-lifting program so that you never work the same muscle group two days in a row. With cardio-exercises, alternate hard days with easy days.

12. **To add variety to your workouts, mix up the methods you use by trying the variations.** Try working the muscle with a standing or sitting alternative. Use dumbbells instead of a bar bell. Try machines instead of free weights. Each will work the muscle in a different way. This helps avoid adaptation.

13. **Embrace cross-training principles.** Repeating the same activity day after day increases your risk for overuse injuries. If you jog one day, on the next day choose an activity that involves your upper body, such as swimming or rowing. Make sure your overall program includes a balance of strength, cardiovascular and flexibility exercises.

14. **Check form and monitor progress by using a mirror.** If you can see the area being worked you will work it harder and with better form.

15. **Wear comfortable clothes that move with you.** They should allow you to see the areas being worked. Breathable fabrics work best. Consider light layers in colder weather. Also wear good-fitting sneakers when doing exercise of any kind.

16. **Large muscles should NOT be worked two days in a row.** They need time for repair. (This is when muscles have been fatigued, not through casual movements).

17. **Abdominal muscles and calves can be worked every day.** They tolerate frequency and repair quickly due to constant use.

18. **Use proper equipment.** *If* you advance to heavy weights you should get some lifting gloves, the kind with no fingertips, to protect hands from calluses. Use a lifting belt if lifting heavy weights on a barbell (squats, etc.). Most gyms have one you can borrow.

19. **Balance your weight training routine with cardiovascular exercise and a healthy diet.** This basic fundamental will yield the greatest benefits from your efforts.

20. **Eat smart.** Maximize results by fueling your body to burn more fat. Choose carbohydrates before workouts and protein after them.

Benefits of Weight-Bearing Exercise

- **Causes the bones to strengthen and stay firm.** It can stop or reverse the bone loss associated with aging. (Osteoporosis).

- **Helps to work joints through a full range of motion**, keeping them strong and flexible, thus improving balance.

- **Helps relieve arthritis** by using the joints and increasing flexibility.

- **Improves the symptoms of many chronic health issues** such as fibromyalgia and chronic fatigue syndrome.

- **Slows the decline of cardio endurance.** Endurance and muscle strength declines progressively after age 30.

- **Can improve total blood cholesterol** and triglyceride levels, decrease blood sugar and improve other risk factors for disease.

- **Can help reduce blood pressure** when used with other healthy behaviors.

- **Can lower cholesterol and help the heart function better** by delivering more oxygen to the cells. It also improves circulation.

- **Can reduce the look of cellulite** by firming up the muscle under the skin and by shrinking some of the fat cells in those areas.

- **Decreases body size by reducing inches.** Muscle weighs more than fat, but takes up less space.

- **Adds variety to your fitness routine** and creates different challenges for your body.

- **Builds lean muscle tissue. This increases metabolism,** which means you burn more calories throughout the day.

- **Increases strength,** which makes everything you do a little easier. This effect will be noticed in many unexpected areas of your life.

- **Strengthens connective tissue, ligaments and tendons**—that keep your body moving.

- **Helps protect your body during movement** and makes you less likely to experience body mechanics injuries.

- **Keeps athletes strong and helps them avoid injuries.** Training specific to a certain sport can help improve power, strength and speed.

- **Allows joints to be better cushioned and protected** during impact activities like walking.

- **Speeds the healing of bone and muscle injuries** and improve the overall quality of life. It is incorporated into many physical therapy rehabilitation plans.

- **Improves posture and overall appearance** by toning and sculpting the muscles.

- **Releases endorphins into the bloodstream that make us feel good.** (Nature's morphine pump).

- **Increases feelings of well-being** and improves body image. As people grow stronger and notice changes, such as being able to lift more weight and body shaping, they build self-confidence.

Get REAL Factoids

1. **Through "purposeful movement" exercise can be incorporated in your lifestyle.** Regular activity can become a way of living, not something you have to schedule time for.

2. **Muscle is more metabolically active than fat.** Even though muscle doesn't burn a huge number of calories on its own, it is still very important for weight loss. A pound of muscle burns more fat and calories than a pound of fat. Muscle increases your average daily metabolic rate which is the foundation for losing fat.

3. **Muscle is heavier than fat, but it takes up less space.** You may see bigger changes in your size and shape than you do in your weight. Muscle and fat are different. Muscle cannot become fat or fat become muscle.

4. **Resistance training can reduce the look of cellulite** by firming up the muscle under the skin and by shrinking some of the fat cells in those areas.

5. **Fat cells cannot be reduced in number but they can be reduced in size.** Fat cells fill up and once they reach capacity they must create *more* fat cells to make space for needed fat storage. Once you have them, you are stuck with them. Your best plan is to not allow your body to store excess calories as fat—which keeps the size of the fat cells reduced. This is managed through your intentional eating methods. To reduce the amount of fat stored in the fat cells you must burn more calories than take in at a given time. This is a reason to avoid overeating at one sitting.

6. **Men have more enzymes for the release of fat.** Men also have about 40 percent more muscle cells than women. The greater

number of muscle cells you have, the more calories will be burned and less stored. This accounts for smaller fat cells.

7. **Women have more enzymes that facilitate the storage of fat.** This is fueled by estrogen and accounts for larger fat cells.

8. **Regular aerobic activity stimulates the enzymes needed for the release of fat.** When people engage in aerobic exercise regularly, they turn on their fat burning mechanisms. Aerobic means "with oxygen" and a constant supply of oxygen is needed for the release of fat. Moderate exercise gives you a steady, increased heart rate and a steady supply of oxygen to your fat cells. This is your fat burning zone.

9. **Aerobic exercise involves your major muscle groups**—such as the buttocks and thighs—in a rhythmical, non-stop movement. This type of movement will elevate the heart rate for an extended period of time.

10. **Anaerobic exercise such as those seen in many sports, stimulate muscle mass and metabolism.** They are not significant for fat releasing because the stop and start movements are not continuous. They do not produce a *steady* increase in heart rate and breathing rate. They are good for overall health.

11. **The average person produces gains** of about three to five pounds of muscle mass every three to four months of regular resistance training. This is affected by your genetics, gender, exercise program and diet. As a result, each person will have a different response to training.

12. **The average woman does not *bulk-up* from strength training** because she does not have the amount of hormones (testosterone) necessary to build massive amounts of muscle.

13. **Trying to gain muscle takes just as much work as losing fat for both men and women.** You will need to continually work your muscles to build and maintain your tone and strength.

14. **Average number of bent-leg push-ups (PU) for women:** (Age 17-19) 11-20 PU, (Age 20-29) 12-22 PU, (Age 30-39) 10-21 PU, (Age 40-49) 8-17 PU, (Age 50-59) 7-14 PU, (Age 60-65) 5-12 PU.

15. **Average number of push-ups (PU) for men:** (Age 17-19)19-34 PU, (Age 20-29) 17-29 PU, (Age 30-39) 13-24 PU, (Age 40-49) 11-20 PU, (Age 50-59) 9-17 PU, (Age 60-65) 6-16 PU.

Resistance Training Methods

Commonly people train using straight sets. They do specified number of repetitions for a specified number of sets, with a rest in between. This is good for the beginning exerciser. Trying other methods periodically will allow the body to work in a new way. By periodically challenging the body with new methods you can keep the results coming. Some other basic options are **super sets, tri sets, circuits and pre-exhaustion.**

Get REAL Note: If during exercise you feel faint, short of breath or have chest pains, stop immediately and seek help.

Super sets: 2 to 3 sets completed *without* a rest in between.

Tri-sets: perform **three different exercises** for the same muscle group **without a rest** in between sets.

Example: Lateral raises, front raises and upright rows (shoulders).

Circuits: completing and combining a series of exercises one after another without a rest. This can also create a cardiovascular workout.

Example: squats with kick backs, Lunge with overhead press, calf raises with bicep curls.

Pre-exhaustion: Working the larger muscle groups first so that you pre-exhaust them, allows the smaller groups to work independently without help from the larger muscles.

Get REAL Note: For week one you will choose a weight that you can perform 8 to 12 repetitions with *proper form.* At the end of that set, your muscle should feel fatigued but not sore or strained. Adjust the amount of weight used until you find the right balance. Remember—you may need to use different amounts of weight for each muscle group or exercise. You can follow a resistance training plan that gradually progresses as you become stronger. Next is an *example* of this type of exercise progression.

Weekly Resistance Training Progression

Week One
1 set of 10 repetitions

Week Two
2 sets of 8 repetitions

Week Three
2 sets of 10 repetitions

Week Four
2 sets of 12 repetitions

Week Five (increase weights)
3 sets of 10 repetitions

Week Six
3 sets of 12 repetitions

Maintenance

Increase weight to meet 2 sets of 10 repetitions or try **Tri-Sets**:

- Circuits of three 1 set of 10 (same muscle group) exercises
- One set (single exercise) followed by one set of the next exercise with no rest in between
- *Example:* Lateral raises, front raises and upright rows (shoulders)
- Repeat the *circuit* of three sets

Routine for Various Fitness Machines

Body part worked:	Name of machine to use:
Chest:	Chest press Machine Fly Machine
Shoulders:	Overhead or Shoulder Press Incline Press
Triceps:	Triceps Press Triceps Extension Lat Pull-Down—Triceps Pull-Downs
Bicep:	Arm Curl Arm Extension
Back:	Lat Pull-Down—Behind Neck Pull-Down Pull Over Back Extension Row
Abdominal:	Abdominal Machine Incline Bench - Crunches
Hip/Thigh:	Hip Abduction Hip Adduction Multi Hip
Legs/Glutes:	Leg Press for Quads and Glutes Leg Extension for Quads Leg Curl for Hamstrings A Step for Lunges (Legs and Glutes)
Calves:	Calve Extension Machine

Sample Warm Up

- Stand with feet shoulder width apart
- Inhale as you bring arms up
  - Grasp hands above head and stretch up
  - Stretch side to side using waist (4-6 times)
- Lower arms to shoulder level
  - Hands are pointed out and arms are parallel to the floor
  - Stretch to right side using the waist and hold
  - Stretch to left side using the waist and hold (repeat 4-6 times)
- Drop arms to side
  - Shoulder shrugs up and down (4-6 times)
- Front neck rolls (gently side to side 4-6 times)
- Take right hand and touch left ear
  - Pull head to the right gently stretching the neck (hold 5 counts)
  - Repeat with left side
- Roll shoulders forward (4-6 times)
- Roll shoulders back (4-6 times)
- Touch hands front to back—back to front (4-6 times)
  - Step, touch (feet together) to the right—repeat to the left (4-6 times)
- Spread legs slightly wider than shoulder width
  - Put hands on knees
  - Pulse side to side by bending knees (left then right) (4-6 times)
  - Knees do not go past toes (feel the pull in the upper legs)
- Plant right foot, lean to that side
  - Bend left knee, pulling foot up toward bottom
  - Straighten leg and plant left foot, repeat series with left leg
  - Optional— bicep curl ups at same time (4-6 times)

- Turn to center
  - Pivot turn by 45 degrees to the right
  - Raise both hands into air as your lunge forward onto right leg
  - Left heel will rise (4-6 times)
  - Bring arms down and pivot opposite side
  - Repeat action onto left leg
  - Right heel will rise (4-6 times)
- Return to the center; bring arms down and feet flat
  - Bend forward with a flat back
  - Arch (like a cat) roll back up slowly Repeat (4-6 times)

Get REAL Resistance Training Menu

Get REAL Note: EC=Extra Challenge Option

CHEST

- Chest Press
- Dumbbell Fly
- Pec Deck
- EC-Push Ups

SHOUDERS

- Lateral Raises
- Front Raises
- Upright Rows
- EC-Shoulder Press

TRICEPS

- Dumbbell Kickback
- Press Downs
- One or Two-Arm Overhead Extensions
- EC-Dips

BICEPS

- Supported Angle Dumbbell Curl
- Double Dumbbell Curls (splits or together)
- Hammer Curls
- EC-Push Ups

BACK

- Lawn Mowers
- Bent-Over Row
- Seated Dumbbell Row
- Bent-Over Fly or Dead Lift
- EC-Superman

ABDOMINALS

- Legs Up Crunch
- 3 Way Slow Crunch
- Double Knee or Bicycle Crunch
- Legs Up – Oblique Twist Crunch
- EC- Side Crunch, Leg Curl Up or Isometric

LEGS, HIPS & BUTTOCKS

- Squats/Plies or Lunges (Alternate or do both)
- Elbows and Knees Series
- Core Floor Series
- EC-Standing Floor Routine

CALVES

- Calves Series (Non-Weighted and Weighted)

(The following worksheets may be downloaded from www.getrealwellnesssolutions.com)

"Build Your Own" Exercise Log

Day 1   Day 2

CHEST	Set/Rep	Wt.	LEGS	Set/Rep	Wt.
SHOULDER	Set/Rep	Wt.	BACK	Set/Rep	Wt.
TRICEPS (Back of arm)	Set/Rep	Wt.	BICEPS (Front of arm)	Set/Rep	Wt.
ABDOMINALS	Set/Rep	Wt.	ABDOMINALS	Set/Rep	Wt.
CALVES	D-1	D-2	CALVES	D-1	D-2

2 Day FULL BODY Home WORKOUT LOG

DAY 1

CHEST	Set/ Rep	Wt.
Chest Press		
Dumbbell Fly		
Pec Deck		
Push Up		
SHOULDERS	Set/ Rep	Wt.
Side Laterals		
Front Raises		
Upright Rows		
Overhead Press		
TRICEPS (Back of arm)	Set/ Rep	Wt.
Dumbbell Kickback		
One-Arm Overhead Extension		
Two-Arm Overhead Extension		
Dips		
ABDOMINALS	Set/ Rep	Wt.
Legs Up Crunch		
3 Way Slow Crunch		
Double Knee or Bicycle Crunches		
Legs Up—Oblique Twist		
CALVES	Rt.	Lt.
Toes Parallel		
Toes In		
Toes Out		
Weighted		

DAY 2

LEGS	Set/ Rep	Wt.
Squats/Plies		
Lunges		
Inner/Outer Leg Lifts Thigh Blasters		
Elbow/Knees Series		
BACK	Set/ Rep	Wt.
Lawn Mowers-One-Arm Rows		
Bent-Over Rows		
Seated Rows		
Bent-Over Fly		
BICEPS (Front of arm)	Set/ Rep	Wt.
Supported Angle Curl Ups		
Double Dumbbell Curls		
Hammer Curls		
Push Up		
ABDOMINALS	Set/ Rep	Wt.
Legs Up Crunch		
3 Way Slow Crunch		
Double Knee or Bicycle Crunches		
Legs Up—Oblique Twist		
CALVES	Rt.	Lt.
Toes Parallel		
Toes In		
Toes Out		
Weighted		

271

2 Day FULL BODY Gym WORKOUT LOG

DAY 1

CHEST	Set/Rep	Wt.
*Bench Press		
*Incline/Decline Dumbbell Fly		
*Incline Dumbbell Press		
Pec Deck Fly or *Pec Deck Machine		
Push Up		

SHOULDERS	Set/Rep	Wt.
Side Laterals		
Front Raises		
Upright Rows		
Overhead Press		
*Dumbbell Rear Laterals		

TRICEPS (Back of arm)	Set/Rep	Wt.
Dumbbell Kickback		
Overhead Extension (One or Two Arm)		
*Cable Press Down		
Dips		
DAILY		

ABDOMINALS	D-1	D-2
Crunches (Options)		
Double Knee Crunch		
Leg Curl Up Crunch		
Side Crunches (Options)		

DAY 2   *Gym Only Addition

LEGS	Set/Rep	Wt.
Squats		
Lunges		
*Outer Leg Raise (Cables) Inner Leg Cross		
*Leg Extension Machine		
*Hamstring Curl Machine		
*Leg Press Machine		

BACK	Set/Rep	Wt.
Lawn Mowers (One-Arm Row)		
Bent-Over Row		
*Seated Pulley Rows		
*Wide Grip Pull-Down		
*Pull Ups		

BICEPS (Front of arm)	Set/Rep	Wt.
Single Dumbbell Curl (Options)		
*Seated Incline Dumbbell Curls		
*Standing Barbell Curl		
*Cable Pull Up		
DAILY		

CALVES	D-1	D-2
Toes Parallel		
Toes In		
Toes Out		
DATE		

Get REAL Basic Exercises

CHEST

Instructions:

- Choose two to three exercises
- Rest 24 hours before working this area again
- Follow with shoulder and triceps exercises

> **Get REAL Trainers Note**: Never overlook the chest and upper body when building lean muscle. This area responds quickly to exercise and can totally change your posture, strength and how you look.

The Chest Press (A classic chest toner!)

- Lay flat on your back.
- Use a step, bench or the floor
  - Arms out to the sides to form a (t)
- Take a dumbbell in each hand
- Bend elbows up to form a 90-degree angle
  - Hands in the air with palms forward
- Press dumbbells up by straightening the arms above your head
  - Be sure to squeeze chest during this movement
  - Focus on a spot on the ceiling and keep your eyes there

- Pause, feel the squeeze and slowly lower the dumbbells
  - Watch form—elbows are bent 90 degrees in starting position
- Return to the starting position
  - Do not "cheat" arms in
  - This is one rep

Gym Alternative:
Bench Press on spotter stand/weight bench using barbell.

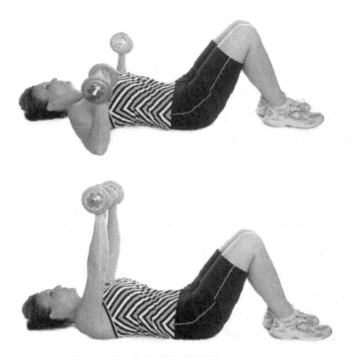

GOAL: Firmer chest with noticeable cleavage line. Increases chest and upper body strength.

Dumbbell Fly

- Lay flat on your back
  - Arms out to the side to form a (t)-palms are up
- Bend elbows (soft elbow-arms still extended) hands are slightly raised
- Take a dumbbell in each hand—palms up
- Squeeze with your chest as you bring dumbbells together over head
  - Focus on a spot on the ceiling and keep your eyes there
  - Watch form—this is a controlled movement
- Pause and feel the squeeze
- Slowly return to the starting position
  - Keep elbows soft and do not lock them
  - This is one rep

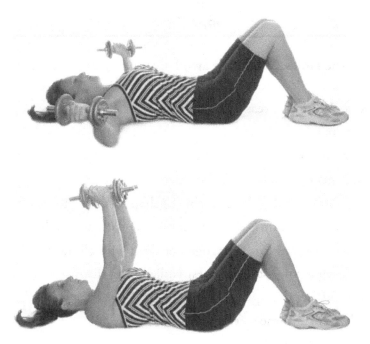

GOAL: Firmer chest and bust line, also works arms and shoulders.

Gym Alternative: *Incline Fly on incline bench.

*Decline Fly on decline bench.

Chair Alternative:
- Sit in chair with arms out to side to form a (t)—palms forward
- Take a dumbbell in each hand
- Bring arms together at shoulder level
    - Keep arms straight with elbows soft
- Pause and feel the squeeze in the chest
- Slowly return to the starting position

Get REAL Trainers Note: Great for the chest, shoulders, upper back and neck! Consider using lighter weights to avoid strain on the neck and upper back.

Note for the ladies: Works the awful area that hangs over the bra!

Pec Deck (Pectoral Press or Butterfly)
- Sit on chair
- Take a dumbbell in each hand
- Raise arms to parallel with shoulders
- Bend elbows 90 degrees to form (L) shape—palms forward
    - Keep upper arms (elbow to shoulder) flat and parallel to floor
- Bring elbows and forearms together (lead with elbows)
    - Watch form—squeeze chest while doing the movement
- Pause and feel the squeeze
- Slowly return to the starting position
    - This is one rep

Gym Alternative: *Pec Deck Machine- sit on bench, place arms behind the pads, press padded bars together using forearms. Keep back pressed into bench.

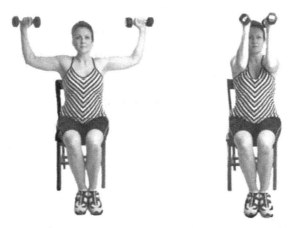

GOAL: Firmer chest/cleavage line, also works arms, shoulders and upper back.

Get REAL Trainers Note: For an abdominal challenge, utilize the Ab Angle- the exercise is done while leaning back at a 45 degree angle or into an exercise ball, using the abdominal muscles to support you.

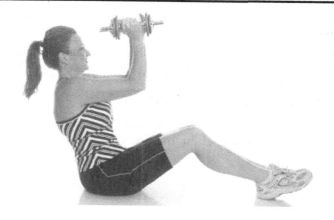

Wall Push Up
(Multi-Functional Upper Body Exercise)

- Stand arms length from the wall
- Place hands shoulder distance apart on the wall
- Lower yourself to the wall using only your arms
- Press yourself back to starting position using only your arms
  - Keep back flat and straight
- This is the most versatile option available!

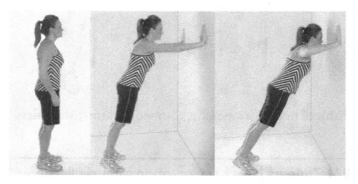

Variations: Arms close together or arms wide apart

Floor Variations: Lay on stomach and back remains flat/straight

Floor Leg Positions:

- Beginner/Easy: Keep knees directly under body
- Female/Moderate: Legs extended and knees remain on ground
- Male/Challenge: full military push up with legs fully extended–advanced, requires greatest core strength

GOAL: A toned upper body, chest and arms.

Traditional Push Up

- Place hands at shoulder level, a hand distance from the shoulder
- Rise up by extending the arms only
    - Keep the back flat and straight
- Pause and feel the tension in the arms and chest
- Slowly lower to the starting position, slightly off the floor
    - This is one rep

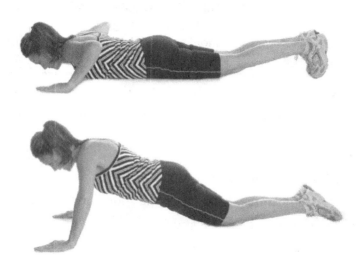

GOAL: Increased upper body strength and tone.

SHOULDERS

Instructions:

- Choose two to three exercises
- Rest 24 hours before working this area again
- Follow with triceps exercises

Get REAL Trainers Note: Never overlook the shoulders and upper body when building lean muscle. This area responds quickly to exercise and promotes good posture. Sculpted shoulders define your shape and make the waist look smaller.

CAUTION: When choosing weights to work this area, consider that the neck area will also be engaged. Strain can result if weight is too heavy.

Side Laterals

- Stand with arms down to your side
    - Use good posture—head, neck and shoulders relaxed
    - Keep back straight and abs tucked in
- Take a dumbbell in each hand, palms face you
- Raise both arms out to the side
    - Keep arms parallel with your shoulders (T-Position)
    - Watch form—arms should be parallel to the floor
    - Do not bunch neck or shoulders
- Pause and feel the squeeze in the shoulder and upper arm
- Slowly return to the starting position
    - This is one rep

Gym Alternative: *****Dumbbell Rear Laterals-** lay belly down on a bench. Weights are held under the bench—raise weights out to sides. Works the back and shoulders.

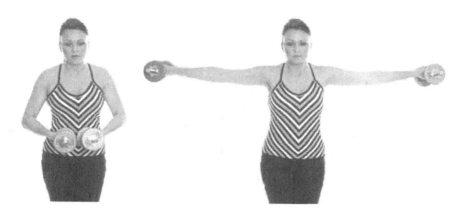

> **<u>Get REAL Trainers Note</u>:** Neck strain is a signal to use lighter weights or to do fewer reps.

GOAL: Shapely toned shoulders with good definition, also tones the upper arm.

Front Raises

- Stand with arms at your side
- Take a dumbbell in each hand, palms to the rear
- Raise both arms straight up (out away from body) until parallel with shoulder
- Watch form—keep arms straight out
  - Body should be relaxed but held in proper posture
  - Do not bunch neck or shoulders
  - NOTE: This could indicate the need for lighter weights or fewer reps
- Pause and feel the squeeze in the shoulder and upper arm
- Slowly lower arms to the starting position
  - This is one rep
  - May do together or in splits (one arm at a time, alternating)

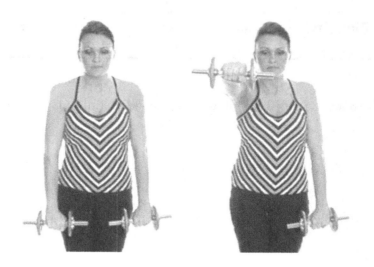

GOAL: A toned and defined shoulder while adding definition to upper arms.

Upright Rows

- Stand with arms straight down in front of you
  - Palms touching the thighs
- Take a dumbbell in each hand and place end to end
- Pull the dumbbells up the body until under the chin
  - Elbows are high and out to the side
  - Keep the dumbbells close together during the raise
  - Watch form—do not scrunch neck or shoulders
  - Keep the proper posture and body relaxed
- Pause and feel squeeze in shoulders, upper arm, upper back and neck
- Slowly lower dumbbells to starting position
  - This is one rep

Get REAL Note: Sore neck may indicate need for lighter weights or fewer reps—always value *quality* over *quantity*.

Variation: May use weighted ball, barbell or broom in place of dumbbells. Keep hands close together during the exercise, a hands distance between them.

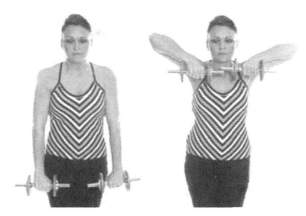

GOAL: Toned and defined shoulder while adding definition to upper back, neck and upper arms.

Overhead Press

- Sit on chair
- Take a dumbbell in each hand
- Raise arms to parallel with shoulders, palms up
- Bend elbows up 90 degrees to form (L) shape—turn palms forward
    - Keep upper arms (elbow to shoulder) flat and parallel to floor
- Raise arms straight above head
- Pause and feel the tension
- Slowly return to the starting position
    - Maintain 90 degree angle—keep arms up in good form
    - This is one rep

Gym Alternative: *Incline Press-same mechanics done on the incline bench (shown).

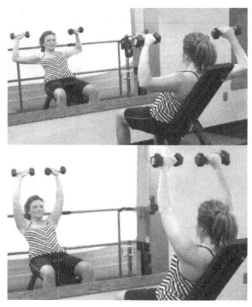

GOAL: Toned and defined shoulder while adding definition to upper back, neck and upper arms.

Chest and Shoulder Stretch

- Sit in chair
- Lean forward
- Reach back with one arm
- Grab chair
- Lean shoulder forward
  - Count 4 full seconds
- Take a deep cleansing breath and release
- Then roll shoulder back
  - Count 4 full seconds
- Take a deep cleansing breath and release
- Repeat with other arm

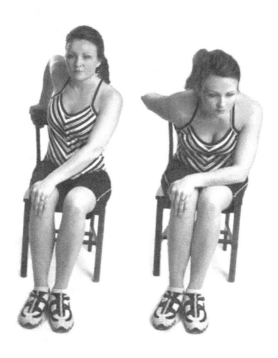

TRICEPS

Instructions:

- Choose two to three exercises
- Rest 24 hours before working this area again
- Follow with biceps exercises if going on, or abdominals

> **Get REAL Trainers Note:** Never overlook triceps. This area responds quickly to exercise and promotes balance and strength. Toned arms define your body and reveal a fit and sculpted shape.

LADIES: This is the area that keeps on waving, long after you stopped! Remember to really work this area. Heavier weights can usually be used.

Dumbbell Kickback (Classic arm-flab toner)

- Sit in a chair holding a dumbbell in your right hand
- Lean forward slightly with you back flat, not arched
- Bend elbow until forearm is parallel with the ground (starting position)
- Press the dumbbell back by extending the elbow fully
  - KEY to this exercise and all triceps work:
  - Upper arm (shoulder to elbow) does not move
  - All motion takes place at the elbow
- Pause and feel the squeeze in the back of the arm—important
- Slowly return to the starting position
  - Resist both ways and go slow
  - Keep arm close to body—quality over quantity
  - This is one rep
- Continue with same arm until set complete
- Then switch arms and repeat the above

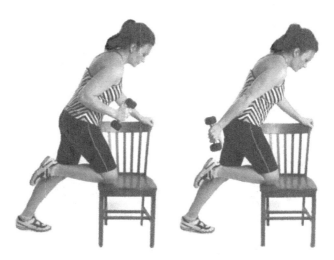

GOAL: A toned and defined back of the arm—Bye-Bye *"batwings!"*

Press Downs

- Stand with dumbbells placed end to end at abdomen level
  - Arms bent 90 degrees
- Press back both arms simultaneously using kick back technique
  - Upper arm (shoulder to elbow) does not move
  - All motion takes place at the elbow
- Pause and feel the squeeze in the back of the arm—important
- Slowly return to the starting position
  - Resist both ways and go slow
  - Keep arms close to body—quality over quantity
  - This is one rep
  - May be done together or in splits (one arm at a time, alternating)

Gym Alternative: *Cable Press Down*-Use *Rope* or *V-attachment* on the overhead pulley system. With elbows tight at sides, press down and slowly release up to start position at the waist.

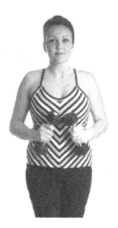 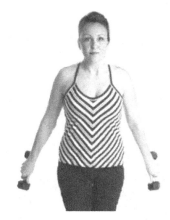

GOAL: A toned and defined back of the arm with no jiggle-jiggle.

Two-Hand Overhead Extension

- Lie on your back (may use bench, step or on the floor)
- Take one dumbbell with both hands—palms together
- Raise arms so that hands are directly above head with elbows bent
  - Dumbbells are close to floor but not touching
  - Elbows are close to head and remain so
  - Note: This is the starting position
- Extend forearm up at the elbow
  - Upper arm (shoulder to elbow) does not move (as always)
  - All movement is in the elbow only
- Pause and feel the squeeze in the back of the arm
- Slowly return to the starting position
  - This is one rep

Variation: Sitting in chair with arms in same position and same technique (shown).

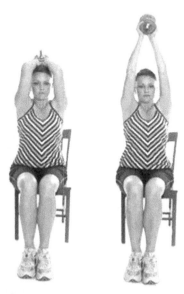

GOAL: A toned and defined back of the arm—no more flabby hangers!

One-Arm Overhead Extension

- Sit in a chair
- Take a dumbbell in your right hand
- Raise your right arm straight up in the air
- Bend your elbow behind your head
  - Note: This is the starting position
- Extend forearm up at the elbow
- Stabilize the active arm with the inactive hand
  - Upper arm (shoulder to elbow) does not move (as always)
  - All movement is in the elbow only
- Pause and feel the squeeze in the back of the arm
- Slowly return to the starting position
  - Keep arm close to the head at all times
  - This is one rep (Continue with same arm until set complete then switch arms)

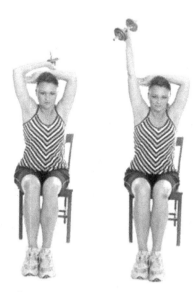

GOAL: A toned back of the arm that doesn't keep waving when you have stopped!

Dips (Most versatile choice)

- Sit on the edge of a chair
- Place your hands beside your hips on the front corner edges
- Slide feet forward (choose your variation)
    - Position feet to reduce strain on the elbows
- Slide your bottom off the chair and dip down into a squat
    - You should feel the work in the back of the arms
    - Do not cheat with legs
    - Use arms only to raise and lower
- Rise back up by straightening the arms
    - This is one rep

Variation: Keep knees directly under you at a 90 degree angle-easiest (shown).

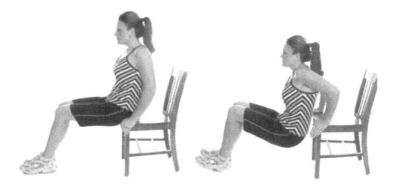

Variation: Can do **one arm dip** the same way. It is a more intense targeting of the muscle more difficult and advanced move.

Advanced Variation: Can rest feet on another bench and repeat the exercise.

GOAL: Great arms with NO back jiggle.

Variation: Can bring **legs straight out** in front of you, either crossed at the ankle or not. This is a more advanced move (shown).

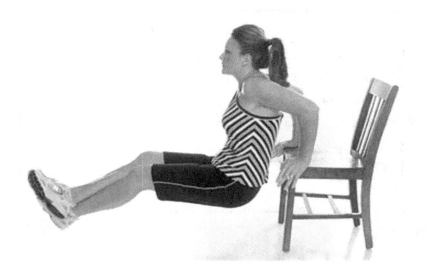

Triceps Stretch

- Raise right arm straight up above head
- Bend elbow behind head
- Grab right hand with left hand and gently pull down
- Feel the stretch in the back of the arm
  - Hold 4 full counts
- Take a deep cleansing breath and release
- Repeat on the other arm

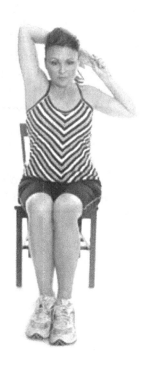

BICEPS

Instructions:

- Choose two to three exercises
- Rest 24 hours before working this area again
- Follow with abdominal or leg exercises, depending on your daily split

Get REAL Trainers Note: Biceps are the muscle group that most think of when you say "make a muscle." Men spend time on this area because of its growth potential (due to their hormonal make-up). Women need to train this area in order to balance the triceps muscle and further define the arms. Women will not "bulk up" due to lack of the male hormones that allow that. Increased arm strength is important when performing daily functions and as a person ages. It keeps bones strong and joints flexible. Most people can use **heavier weight** for this muscle.

Supported Angle Dumbbell Curl
(Good start—aides control)

- Sit in chair and bend forwards slightly
- Hold dumbbell in right hand with palm up
- Place right elbow into *the inside* of the right knee for support
- Extend forearm to line up with lower leg
- Fully bend elbow
  - This is a controlled movement
  - Resist up and down
- Pause and feel the squeeze in the upper arm
  - Note: All action is in the elbow only
  - Key: Upper arm (shoulder to elbow) does not move
- Extend elbow slowly to starting position
  - This is one rep
- Continue on same side until set complete then switch arms

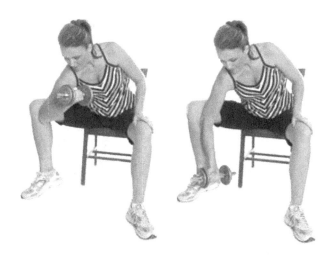

GOAL: A toned and balanced upper arm, also adds strength and definition.

Dumbbell Curl (Classic Single)

- Sit in chair or stand
- Extend right arm along side
- Hold dumbbell in right hand with palm up
- Fully bend elbow
  - This is a controlled movement
  - Resist up and down
- Pause and feel the squeeze in the upper arm
  - May place left hand under elbow for support
  - **Note: All action is in the elbow only**
  - **Key:** Upper arm (shoulder to elbow) **does not** move
- Extend elbow slowly to starting position
  - This is one rep
- Complete the set then change arms and repeat

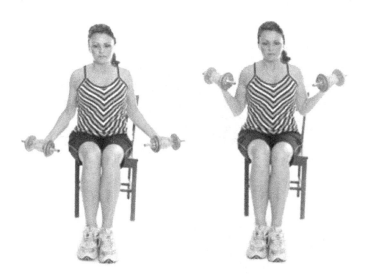

GOAL: A toned and defined front of the arm, in balance with triceps.

Variations:

Double Dumbbell Curls- are same as above except you bend both elbows up at the same time (shown).

Split curls- are done on one side then the other.

Broom or Barbell Curls- are same as above except you place hands shoulder width apart. Palms up on the broom or barbell and both elbows bend up at the same time.

Gym Alternatives:

* **Incline Dumbbell Curl-** Curls done on incline bench.

*Cable **Pull-Up-** Perform as above using lower pulley cable outlet with long bar attachment.

Hammer Curls
- Sit in chair or stand
- Extend right arm along side
- Hold a dumbbell in each hand with palms **turned in** toward the body
- Fully bend both elbows up at the same time (double)
  - May do **single arm curls, double curls** or **split curls**
  - This is a controlled movement
  - Resist up and down
- Pause and feel the squeeze in the upper arm
  - **Note: All action is in the elbow only**
  - **Key:** Upper arm (shoulder to elbow) **does not** move
- Extend elbow slowly to starting position
  - This is one rep
- Complete the set then change arms and repeat

GOAL: A toned and defined upper arm.

Bicep Stretch

- Take right arm across body horizontally
- Grab right elbow with left hand
- Pull slightly
- Feel the stretch in the arm
  - Hold for 4 full counts
- Take a deep cleansing breath and release
- Repeat with left arm

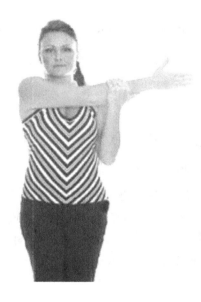

BACK

Instructions:

- Choose two to three exercises
- Rest 24 hours before working this area again
- Follow with leg or bicep exercises, depending on your daily split

Get REAL Trainers Note: The back is used for most daily functions. It can be difficult to isolate and often this fact leads people to overlook it. Balanced back strength will reduce injury and increase your coordination. The back will balance your abdominal core strength and essential to good posture. Most back exercises involve a rowing motion.

Lawn Mowers/One Arm Row

- Stand next to a chair
- Bend so that left hand is touching the chair seat
- Extend right arm straight while holding a dumbbell—palm to body
  - Arms are parallel to each other
- Pull right elbow back and up as if starting a lawn mower
  - Resist up and resist down
  - This is a controlled movement
- Pause and feel the squeeze in the upper back
- Slowly return to the starting position
  - This is one rep
- Continue on same side until set complete then switch arms

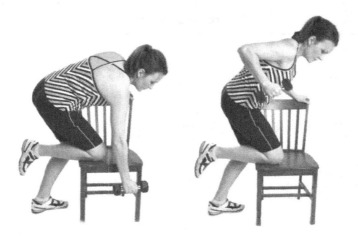

GOAL: A more toned and stronger back. Along with abdominals strengthens core.

Bent-Over Bilateral Row

- Sit on a chair
- Bend forward 45 degrees
- Take a dumbbell in each hand
    - Arms at your side and hanging straight down
- Pull arms up with palms facing in
    - Dumbbells stay close to the body
- Elbows bow out slightly
- Shoulder blades come close together
- Pause and feel that squeeze in the upper back
    - Watch form—don't let posture sag
    - Relax the neck
- Slowly return to the starting position
    - This is one rep

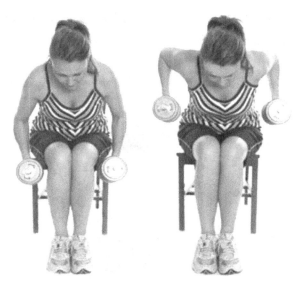

GOAL: A toned and stronger back. Enhances upper back appearance and strength.

Seated Dumbbell Row

- Sit on the floor
- Brace your feet in front of you, shoulder width apart
- Grasp dumbbells with both hands
  - Arms are out and parallel to the floor
- Roll shoulders back and pull ribcage up which arches the back
  - Maintain this upright posture—important
- Slowly pull the dumbbells into your rib cage
  - Keep arms parallel to the floor
  - Dumbbells will be at underarm area
- Pause and feel the squeeze across the back
- Push the dumbbells to the starting position
  - Go slowly and resist both ways
  - This is one rep

Gym Alternatives (Back): *Seated Pulley Row-Perform as above using lower pulley cable outlet with butterfly attachment.

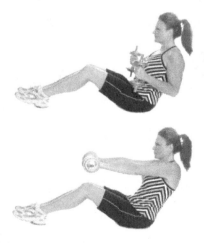

GOAL: A firm and toned back with added strength.

Bent-Over Fly

- Sit on a chair
- Bend forward 45 degrees
- Take a dumbbell in each hand
  - Palms face each other at knee level
- Raise arms up and away from your body until parallel with shoulders
  - Keep elbow soft and extend almost fully at shoulder level
- Pause and feel that squeeze in the upper back
  - Watch form—don't let posture sag
  - Relax your neck
- Slowly return to the starting position
  - This is one rep

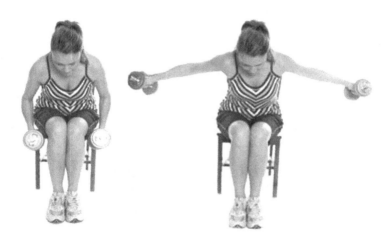

GOAL: A toned and stronger back. Enhances back appearance and strength.

Dead Lift

- Stand straight with proper posture
- Bend at waist and reach down to pick up dumbbells
- Slowly straighten knees but do not lock them
- Pull dumbbells up until you are in a standing and upright position
  - Arms remain straight—palms facing the body
  - Keep the weight close to the body
- Slowly lower weights to the starting position without bending knees
  - This is one rep

Get REAL Note: It may take time to increase flexibility before you can reach the floor.

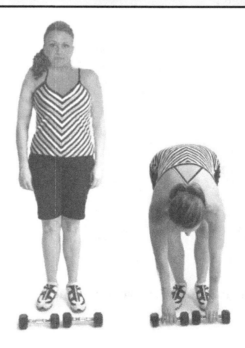

GOAL: A strong back with added flexibility.

Wide Grip Pull Down (Gym Option)

- Sit on the bench in front of the upper pulley cable outlet
- Sit forward on bench
  - Use wide grip bar in the upper attachment
- Brace your feet in front of you and knees comfortably under the pads
- Grasp the wide handles with both hands
- Slowly lower the bar to shoulder level, hands shoulder width apart
- Pause and feel the squeeze across the back
- Return to the starting position—slowly with resistance
  - This is one rep

Superman

- Lay flat on stomach
- Arms straight above head and legs stretched out
- Slowly raise right arm and left leg
  - Hold this for 5 full seconds
- Feel the squeeze in the back area
  - Continue to breathe
- Release arm and leg back to the floor
  - This is one rep
- Repeat with opposite side

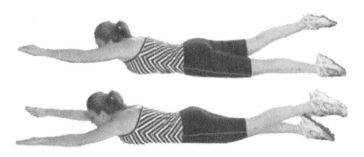

GOAL: Stronger core muscles and back, stretches and strengthens.

Back Stretch

- Sit in a chair
- Bend at the waist
- Arch back and grab inside of the ankles
- Feel the stretch in the back
  - Hold 4 full counts
- Take a deep cleansing breath and release

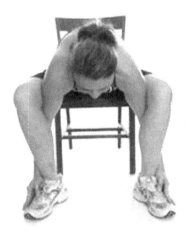

ABDOMINALS

Instructions:

- Choose three to five exercises
- No Rest is required before working this area again
- Work daily alone or in conjunction with other series

<u>**Get REAL Trainers Note**</u>: The abdominal muscle group is used for most daily functions. Balanced core strength will reduce injury and increase your coordination. The abdominal area needs to be in balance with your back. Tight abdominals hold the intestines and internal organs in place. Weak muscles allow the organs to fall forward and protrude out.

Most abdominal muscles are hidden under a layer of fat. Even the tightest muscle—six pack abs—will **never** be seen if that layer of fat is not reduced through weight loss. Your body shape and genetic makeup will determine if you store excess fat in this area. Because of the dangers that fat stored around organs and in the abdominal area pose, a routine of exercise and dietary changes are needed to improve your risk factors.

Crunches (Basic)

- Lie on your back with knees bent or on a chair
- Place hands gently behind head or straight up in the air
  - Pick a spot on the ceiling and keep your eyes there
- Raise shoulders off the ground by contracting the abdominal muscles
  - Keep your chin a fists distance from your chest
  - Keep elbows soft
- Pause and feel the abdominal area tighten
  - Keep low back pressed into the floor
  - Keep breathing
- Slowly lower back to starting position

Get REAL Abdominal Key:

✓ Inhale during extension (when releasing crunch or laying back)
✓ Exhale during contraction (when crunching or bending up

Variation: Decline Crunch- is done on the decline bench with legs over and tucked under the rollers (adds more resistance).

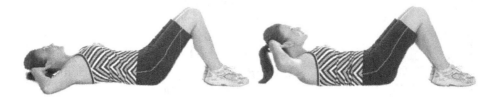

3 Way Slow Crunch

- Place hands gently behind head as above or straight up in the air
- Raise shoulders off the ground by contracting the abdominal muscles
  - Pick a spot on the ceiling and keep your eyes there
- Pause 3 times on the way up to increase the abdominal tightening
  - Keep your chin a fists distance from your chest
  - Keep elbows soft
- Pause and hold five seconds in the highest position
  - Feel the abdominal area tighten
  - Hold the position using only abdominals
  - Keep low back pressed into the floor
- Maintain proper breathing
  - Slowly lower back to starting position in one fluid motion

Legs Up Crunch

- Adjust so that back is flat on mat and in a comfortable position
- Place fingers gently behind ears
  - Pick a spot on the ceiling and keep your eyes there
- Keep your chin a fists distance from your chest
- Raise shoulders off the ground by contracting the abdominal muscles
  - Keep elbows soft and open (do not bring elbows in)
- Pause and feel the abdominal area tighten
  - Keep low back pressed into the floor
  - Keep breathing (Inhale during extension/exhale during contraction)
- Slowly lower shoulders to starting position legs remain elevated throughout

Variation: Alternate raising each leg and tapping down each leg (increases difficulty).

Variations: Multiple variations of abdominal crunches can be done. Mixing up your routine can help you to avoid adaptation to the exercise. Consider balancing on a fitness ball to add greater challenge.

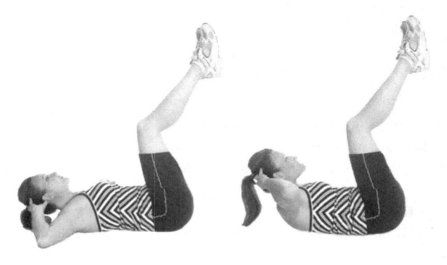

GOAL: Tighter abdominal muscles and a flatter abdomen.

Side Crunch (Oblique Twist)

- Lie on your right side with knees bent
- Place hands gently behind the head
  - Pick a spot on the ceiling and keep your eyes there
- Twist upper body so face is up
- Lift shoulders off the floor by contracting the abdominal muscles
- Pause and feel the tightened abdominal and waist area
- Slowly return to starting position
  - This is one rep
- Continue on this side until set complete
- Then switch sides and repeat

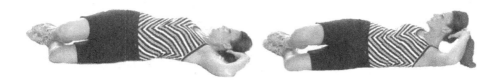

Double Knee Crunch

- Lay on the back with knees bent
- Gently place hands behind the head
  - Pick a spot on the ceiling and keep your eyes there
- Bring knees and elbows together by contracting abdominal muscles
  - Keep a fist distance between chin and chest
  - Keep low back pressed into the floor
- Slowly lower to the starting position
  - Do not let feet touch the ground
  - This is one rep

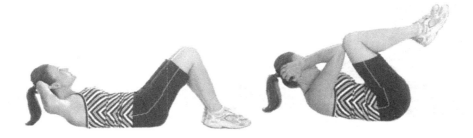

Variation: Frogs

- Place hands on forehead, elbows almost together
- Cross ankles with knees out
- Crunch elbows to the knees
- Use same mechanics as above

Legs Up- Oblique Twist Crunch

- Lie on your back with knees bent and legs raised (May also be done with legs down and bent, or in a 10 reps up and 10 reps down series)
- Cross right foot onto left knee
  - Adjust so that back is flat on mat and in a comfortable position
- Place fingers gently behind ears
- Raise shoulders off the ground by contracting the abdominal muscles, keeping legs raised
  - Keep your chin a fist's distance from your chest
  - Keep elbows soft and open (do not bring elbows in)
  - Pick a spot on the ceiling and keep your eyes there
- Rise up while twisting slightly to the right
- Bring left elbow toward (not touching) the right knee (legs remain elevated)
- Pause and feel the side and abdominal areas tighten
- Return to start position
- Slowly lower shoulders to starting position
  - Keep low back pressed into the floor
  - This is one rep
- Complete set, switch legs and repeat series

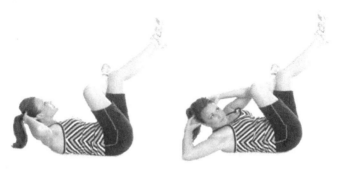

GOAL: Tighter abdominal muscles and a trim waist line.

Bicycle Crunch

- Lie on back with knees bent and legs raised (remain up throughout)
- With legs still elevated, straighten right leg and bring left knee closer
- Take right elbow toward the left knee
- Switch legs by extending the left and bring right knee close
- Take left elbow toward the right knee
    - Keep low back pressed into the floor
    - Keep breathing
    - This is one rep
- Continue to repeat series

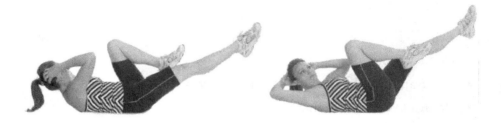

GOAL: Flatter and tighter abs.

Leg Curl Up Crunch (bench)

- Lie back flat on a bench or step
- Legs off the end of the bench or step
    - Pick a spot on the ceiling and keep your eyes there
- Grasp the top of the bench or step with both hands
- Contract abdominal muscles to curl knees up
- Keep small of back pressed into the bench or step at all times
- Pause and feel the squeeze in the abs
- Slowly lower back to the starting position
    - Feet do not touch the floor
    - This is one rep

Variation: can use a medicine ball between the knees for added degree of difficulty and benefit.

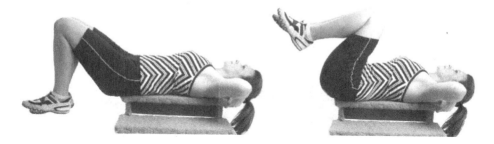

GOAL: Lower abdominal strength and tone.

Leg Curl Up Crunch (floor)

- Lie flat on a back
- Bend knees and lift feet slightly off floor
  - Pick a spot on the ceiling and keep your eyes there
- Place hands under buttocks
- Contract abdominal muscles to curl knees up
- Keep small of back pressed into the floor at all times
- Pause and feel the squeeze in the abs
- Slowly lower back to the starting position
  - Feet do not touch the floor
  - This is one rep

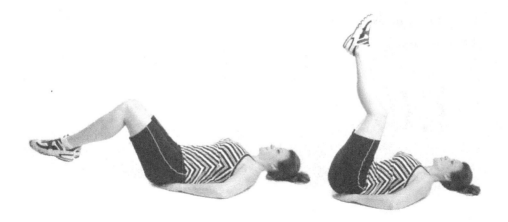

GOAL: Increase abdominal core strength and flatten midsection.

Chair Abdominals

Get REAL Note: You don't have to lay on the floor to increase abdominal strength or flatten your midsection. The key is isolating the core muscles and tensing and releasing them. The following exercises can be done by all fitness levels and in most settings. Focus on using the abdominal muscles to produce the movement. This is a workout!

Abdominals Chair Alternative #1:

- Sit on edge of chair
- Lean back with legs bent in front of you
- Grasp the corners of the chair with both hands
- Contract the abdominal muscle to bring knees up
- Upper back may be pressed into the chair if necessary
- Pause and feel the squeeze in the abs
- Slowly lower back to the starting position
  - Feet do not touch the floor
  - This is one rep

Chair Alternative #2:

- As #1 but instead of just raising knees
- Kick forward slowly—keeping tension in the abdominals
- Return back to start

Chair Alternative #:3

- As #1 but instead of just raising knees
- Kick forward slowly to the right with both legs extended
  - Keep tension in the abdominals
- Return back to start
- Kick forward slowly to the left with both legs extended
  - Keep tension in the abdominals
- Return back to start

Chair Alternative #:4

- Cross arms across chest
- As #1 but instead of just raising knees straight up
- Bring each knee to the opposite elbow
- Return back to start
- Repeat alternating each knee—keeping tension in the abdominals

Isometric Abdominals

Plank (first shown)

- Roll onto stomach
- Raise upper body onto forearms
  - Neck relaxed and face forward
- Rise up on toes—keeping back flat and elbows on mat
- Contract abdominals to hold this pose and feel the abdominal tension
  - Hold 10 full counts or more depending on degree of difficulty
- Take a deep cleansing breath and release

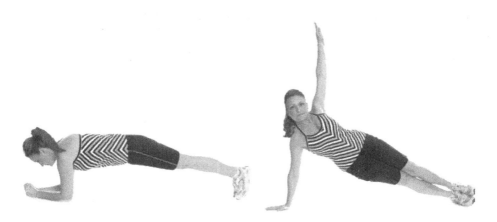

T- Stand (second shown)

- Rise up onto your side
- One hand on the floor and opposite arm mirroring it in the air
- Feet start with one straight and one bent under you
- Kick both legs out straight while maintaining T-position with arms
  - Use your core muscles to maintain this pose for intervals
  - Progress time as you are able to hold position

Variation: T-Stand Twist-

- Take top hand and bend forward at the waist
- Bring the top hand down and through the space under the waist
- Twist back to the original arm extended up position

GOAL: Tighter abdominal muscles and core through isolation and stabilization.

Abdominal Stretch

(first shown)

- Roll onto stomach
- Lie flat with hands up by face
- Raise upper body gently onto forearms
  - Neck relaxed and face forward
- Only rise slightly off the floor
- Feel the abdominal stretch
  - Hold 4 full counts
- Take a deep cleansing breath and release

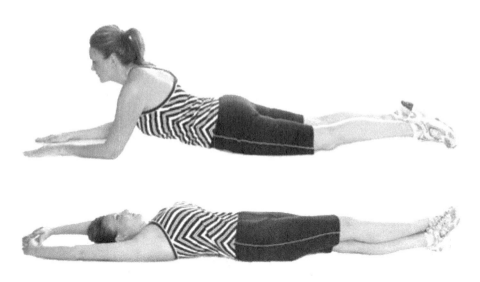

Long Line Stretch

(second shown)

- Lying on back, take arms above head
- Grasp hand and cross ankles
- Stretch long and hold
- Switch ankles and repeat stretch
    - Do not bounce
    - Feel the rib cage rise up out of the abdomen
- Concentrate on breathing fully in and out abdominally

LEGS, HIPS & BUTTOCKS

Instructions:

- Choose three to five exercises (more if working it alone)
- Rest 24 hours before working this area again
- Follow with back exercises if going on or focus on this area alone

Get REAL Trainers Note: Legs are worked regularly when walking and moving. The thighs or quadriceps muscle group make up your biggest muscle area. There are many exercises that target the legs. Mixing up your exercises will prevent boredom and keep your workouts fresh. Utilize exercises that only use your body for resistance to take your leg workouts anywhere.

Working the legs from all angles is important. In this session you will also engage the gluteal muscles (your backside) and your hips. Don't forget the back of the legs—your hamstrings. Choose a variety to maintain balance. Strong legs will propel you faster and improve coordination. Building this lean muscle really burns calories!

Squats (Classic leg and back side exercise)

- Stand with feet shoulder width apart
    - Pick a spot on the wall and focus there
    - Keep chin up and neck relaxed
- Bend knees as if sitting in a chair
    - Buttocks will extend out and back is angled and flat
    - Watch form—DO NOT let knees extend over ankles
- Pause and feel the squeeze in the buttocks and tops of the legs
- Slowly rise back to standing using the legs and tightening the buttocks
    - This is one rep
- Repeat set with legs close together

Gym Alternative: *Weighted-Barbell resting on shoulders, adds difficulty.

Variation: *Sit and taps-Stand in front of a chair. Sit down briefly and then immediately stand back up by squeezing the buttocks and using the larger thigh muscles.

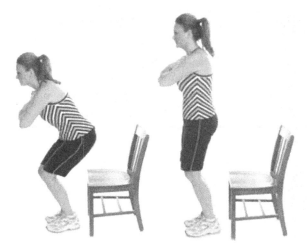

GOAL: Firm, defined legs and back side.

Plies

- With legs in wide stance (greater than hip distance)
- Lower body by bowing knees out to the side
- Pause in the lowered position
  - Do not let knees extend beyond toes
- Squeeze back up using gluteal muscles only

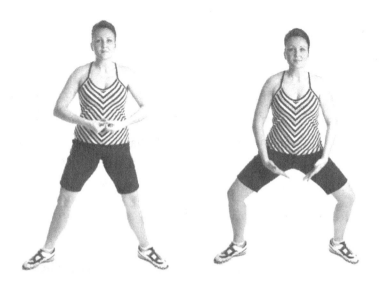

Variation: Rise up onto your toes when returning to the standing position. Squeeze calves and then lower your heel back to the starting position. This adds a multifunctional dimension to the exercise.

GOAL: Firmer and more defined legs and buttocks. Also slims hips and adds leg strength.

Lunges

- Stand with a step in front of you
- Step out putting the whole right foot firmly on the step
- Bend left knee to about step level, thus lowering the body
- Straighten the left knee, rising up to a standing position
- Bring right foot back next to the left
  - Keep upper body with proper posture
  - This is one rep
- Repeat series using the left foot

Variation: Can use dumbbells with arms extended, do bicep curls or overhead presses. The more **arm work** done, the more advanced the move. Master the lunge before adding weights and use the weights for a while before adding the movements. This is more advanced and will save time by targeting two muscle groups at once.

Variation: Reverse lunges can be done by starting on the step and stepping back into the lunge.

Variation: Walking lunges can add difficulty and toning when combined with your routine.

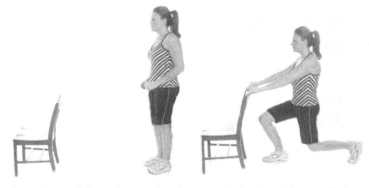

GOAL: A tight and firm buttocks, hips and thighs. This will slim the hip and outer thigh area.

Outer Leg Raise

Floor Core Exercise #1
- Lay on right side with upper body raised on right elbow
- Rotate forward and bring left elbow near the right
  - Right leg slightly bent
- Left leg extended and stacked over right
  - Important—hips are rolled forward
  - Foot is flexed not pointed (lift heel)
- Place left hand on hip to feel area being worked
- Slowly raise left leg, leading with heel and pause
- Pause and feel the squeeze (burning) in the outer hip and thigh area
  - This does not have to be high off the ground to be effective
  - It is a controlled movement
- Slowly lower to the starting position
  - Do not let legs touch, keep top leg slightly elevated
  - Use resistance up and down
  - Quality over quantity
  - This is one rep
- Continue with right leg until set complete then switch legs

Variation: When leg is raised and straight

- Bend at the knee
- Bring knee to floor with foot elevated
- Extend back to straight position (elevated as start)
- Lower to starting position

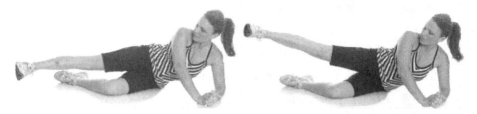

GOAL: Slimming of the hip and outer thigh area.

Outer Leg Lift Chair Alternative:

- Sit with left cheek on the right side of the chair
- Right leg extended to side and straight
- Turn body so that both hands support you on the left side of chair
  - Important—hips are rolled *forward*
  - Foot is flexed not pointed (lift heel)
- Slowly raise right leg leading with heel and pause
- Pause and feel the squeeze (burning) in the outer hip and thigh area
  - This does not have to be high off the ground to be effective
  - It is a controlled movement
- Slowly lower to the starting position
  - Do not let legs touch, keep top leg slightly elevated
  - Use resistance up and down
  - Quality over quantity
  - This is one rep
- Continue with right leg until set complete then switch legs
- Switch to right cheek on left edge of chair and repeat the above

Gym Alternative: *Cable Raise

- Stand facing the cable pulley set at the floor setting
- Put your foot through the leg strap
  - Face so that when raising your leg to the side, you keep the tension
- Raise right leg out to side
- Pause when you feel a squeeze in the hip and buttocks
- Slowly return to the starting position

Inner Leg Lift

Floor Core Exercise #2

- Lay on right side, upper body is propped on right elbow
- Left leg is bent with foot flat and knee up
- Right leg is out slightly and straight with toe flexed, not pointed
- Slowly raise right leg off the floor
  - Lead with the heel using the inner thigh muscles
- Pause and feel the squeeze (burning) in the inner thigh
- Slowly lower the leg to the starting position
  - Do not let leg touch the ground
  - This is one rep
- Continue with right leg until set is complete then switch legs
- Turn onto left side and repeat the above

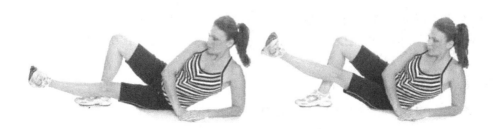

GOAL: Slimming of the hip and inner thigh area.

Inner Leg Lift Chair Alternative:

- Sit forward in the chair
- Right leg down
- Left leg is bent 45 degrees and elevated to the front
  - Left foot is flexed not pointed (raise heel)
- Slowly raise left leg leading with heel and pause
- Pause and feel the squeeze (burning) in the inner thigh area
  - This does not have to be high off the ground to be effective
  - It is a controlled movement
- Slowly lower to the starting position
  - Do not let leg touch the floor
  - Use resistance up and down
  - Quality over quantity
  - This is one rep
- Continue with left leg until set complete then switch legs

Gym Alternative: *Cable Cross

- Stand facing away from the cable pulley set at the floor setting
- Put your foot through the leg strap
  - Face so that when pulling your leg across the body you keep tension in the cable
- Raise leg across your body until you feel tension in the inner thigh
- Pause and feel the squeeze
  - Resist up and down
- Slowly return to the starting position

331

Thigh Blasters

Floor Core Exercise #3

- Sit on floor with right leg bent and left leg straight
- Hug right leg
- Flex left foot
- Raise left leg up (lift heel off floor) until you feel a squeeze in the top of the leg
- Pause and feel the tension
  - Resist up and down
- Return slowly to the starting position
  - This is one rep
- Continue with right leg until set complete then switch legs

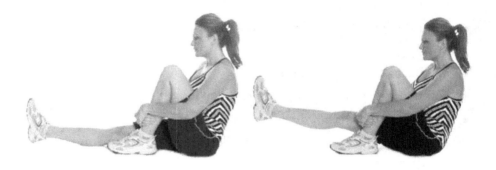

GOAL: Slimmer and firmer thighs. Also tones and strengthens legs.

Thigh Blaster Chair Alternative:

- Sit in chair with right leg bent and left leg straight
  - Right heel can rest on chair or if too difficult against chair leg
- Hug right leg
- Flex left foot
- Raise left leg up (lift heel off floor) until you feel a squeeze in the top of the leg
- Pause and feel the tension
  - Resist up and down
- Return slowly to the starting position
  - This is one rep
- Continue with right leg until set complete then switch legs

Knees and Elbows Series

Floor exercises are done in the "knees and elbows" position with forearms on the mat.

#1 Kick Backs

- Pull knee up to chest
- Then kick leg back raising thigh parallel to ground
    - Leg is bent 90 degrees at the knee and foot is flat
- Pause and feel the stretch in the buttocks and back of the legs
- Return to the starting position, this is one rep
- Repeat with other leg after completing the set

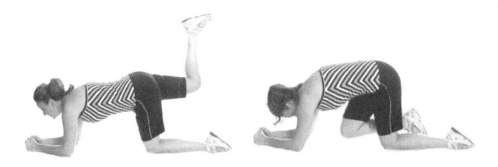

Kick Backs Chair Alternative:

- Sit with left cheek on the right side of the chair
- Right leg is extended to side and bent
- Leg is bent 90 degrees at the knee and foot is above floor
- Turn body so that both hands support you on the left side of chair
    - Important—hips are rolled *forward*
    - Foot is flexed not pointed
- Press right leg to the back, leading with heel and pause
- Pause and feel the squeeze (burning) in the buttocks and outer hip
    - This does not have to be far back to be effective
    - It is a controlled movement
- Slowly bring knee forward to the starting position (knee up/foot down)
    - Use resistance back and forward
    - Quality over quantity
    - This is one rep
- Continue with right leg until set complete then switch legs
- Switch to right cheek on left edge of chair and repeat the above

Knees and Elbows Series continued

#2 Kick Up Press

- Kick leg back raising thigh parallel to ground
  - Leg is bent 90 degrees at the knee and foot is flat
- Raise the thigh up, keeping knee angle and foot into the air
- Pause and feel the stretch in the buttocks and back of the legs
- Return thigh to parallel to floor, this is one rep
- Repeat with other leg after completing the set

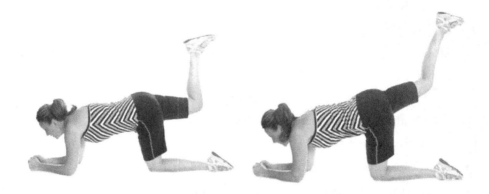

Kick Up Press Chair Alternative:

While doing the Kick Back (See Kick Backs Chair Alternative)

Do short pulses in the press back position (Targets buttocks)

#3 Bad Dogs (Hip Rotation)

- Raise knee straight out to side until entire leg is parallel to ground
  - Knee remains bent at 90 degree angle
- Pause and feel the tension in outer leg
- Return to starting position, this is one rep
- Repeat with other leg after completing the set

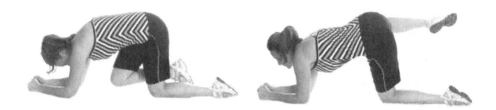

Bad Dogs Chair Alternative:

- Sit with left cheek on the right side of the chair
- Right leg is extended to side and bent
- Turn body so that both hands support you on the left side of chair
  - Important—hips are rolled *forward*
  - Foot is flexed not pointed (Lift heel)
- Slowly raise right knee up and straight out to side until entire leg is parallel to ground
- Knee remains bent at 90 degree angle
- Pause and feel the tension in outer leg
  - This does not have to be high off the ground to be effective
  - It is a controlled movement
- Slowly lower to the starting position
  - Use resistance up and down
  - Quality over quantity
  - This is one rep
- Continue with right leg until set complete then switch legs
- Switch to right cheek on left edge of chair and repeat the above

Variation: When knee is raised and bent, straighten and return to bent position. This adds difficulty.

GOAL: Slimmer, firmer hips and thighs. Also tones and strengthens buttocks.

Hamstring Curl Machine (Gym Option)

- Set appropriate weight
- Lay stomach down on the bench
- Adjust so that the ankles go under rollers
  - Chin is down on the bench throughout
  - Keep the hipbones pressed into the bench at all times
- Slowly pull the rollers up until they touch the buttocks
- Pause in the contracted position
  - Hold for a full 2 counts
- Slowly lower it back to starting position using resistance
  - This is one rep

Leg Extension Machine (Gym Option)

- Set appropriate weight
- Sit on the extension machine
- Adjust so that the ankles go under rollers
  - Keep low back pressed into bench at all times
- Slowly raise the rollers up
- Pause when your legs are straight out in front of you
  - Hold for a full 2 counts
- Slowly lower it back to starting position using resistance
  - This is one rep

Leg Press Machine (Gym Option)

- Set appropriate weight
- Lie or sit on the machine with back flat
  - Keep shoulders back
- Position feet on flat sled with knees bent
- Extend your legs—thus pushing the sled or seat forward
- Pause when your legs are straight out
  - Do not lock knees
  - Hold for a full 2 counts
- Slowly lower to starting position maintaining resistance
  - This is one rep

GOAL: Toned upper legs (quadriceps) and added strength.

Quad and Hamstring Stretch

- Extend right leg out
- Bend forward with hands on right knee or chair back
  - Left leg is back and straight
  - Both feet are flat on the ground
  - Knee does not go beyond toes
- Feel the stretch in the legs
  - Hold 4 full counts
- Take a deep cleansing breath and release
- Bring right leg back slightly
- Flex right toes up and keep right leg straight
- Lean forward and bend left knee out to side while squatting slightly
- Hands on right knee or chair and pull toes up
- Feel the stretch in the back of the right leg
  - Hold 4 full counts
- Take a cleansing breath and release
- Repeat with left leg

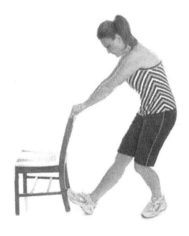

CALVES

Instructions:

• Choose either weighted or non-weighted series (may do both)

• No Rest is required before working this area again

• Work daily alone or in conjunction with other series

Get REAL Trainers Note: The calves are used daily when walking and can be worked daily. Strong calves will balance the look of your legs and provide functional shape. They help propel you when walking and give you a "spring" in your step.

Calve Raises (non-weighted)

- Stand with feet shoulder width apart
  - Maintain proper posture
  - May use a step or not use one
- If using a step, let heels fall off the edge
  - May use a chair or the wall for balance
- FEET PARALLEL
- Rise up onto the balls of the feet
- Pause and feel the squeeze in the back of the lower leg
- Slowly lower back to the starting position
  - This is one rep
- Repeat above with
- TOES POINTED OUT and
- TOES POINTED IN

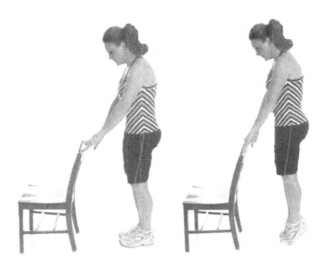

GOAL: Shapely and toned calves.

Calve Raises (weighted)

- Stand with feet shoulder width apart
  - Maintain proper posture
  - May use a step or not use one
- If using a step, let heels fall off the edge
  - May use a chair or the wall for balance
- FEET PARALLEL
- Bend left knee
- Hold a dumbbell in the right hand
- Touch dumbbell to the back of the right leg
- Rise up onto the ball of the right foot
- Pause and feel the squeeze in the back of the lower leg
- Slowly lower back to the starting position
  - This is one rep
- Repeat above switching legs
- Right leg bent/weight behind left leg
- Rise up onto ball of left foot (as above)
- Pause and feel the squeeze in the back of the lower leg
- Slowly lower back to the starting position
  - This is one rep

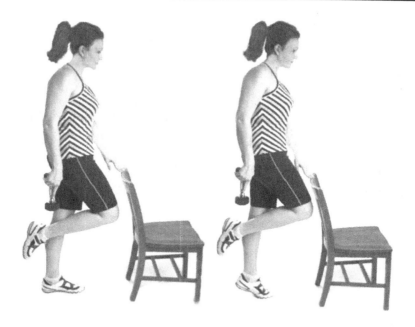

GOAL: Shapely and toned calves.

Calves/Hamstring Stretch

- Lift toes up against a step or the wall
- Feel the stretch in the back of the lower leg
  - Hold 4 full counts
- Bend opposite knee and sit back being supported with the bent leg
- Feel the stretch up the back of the straight leg
- Take a deep cleansing breath and release
- Repeat with other leg

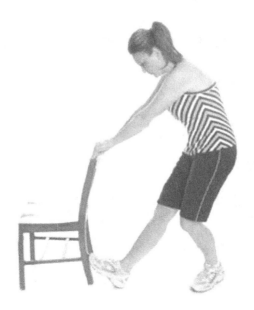

GLOSSARY

(5-HTP): It is an over-the-counter nutrient called 5-hydroxytryptophan. This is the immediate precursor to serotonin, which can also elevate brain serotonin levels.

Ab Angle: Doing an exercise while leaning back at a 45 degree angle or into an exercise ball, using the abdominal muscles to support you.

Abduction: Movement away from the midline of the body.

Adaptation Principle: Your body is smart and can quickly become accustomed or adapted to consistent patterns. It is best to keep your metabolism constantly guessing, which prevents your body from quickly *adapting* to a certain routine of exercise or number of calories it expects to receive. This, in turn, helps keep your metabolism efficient. By not allowing the body to adapt to a regular routine, you force the body to work at a more beneficial level. Changing exercise routines and calorie levels will accomplish this.

Adduction: Movement toward the midline of the body.

Adrenaline: (Epinephrine): A hormone secreted by the adrenal glands, generally under conditions of stress that causes physiologic symptoms.

Aerobic Capacity: This refers to how efficiently your muscles use oxygen and convert fat into fuel. It is increased by regular sustained activity.

Aerobic Exercise: Occurs when any group of large muscles move rhythmically for at *least five minutes* at a sufficient intensity or work level. This should cause the heart rate be consistently elevated. Twenty minutes of sustained activity is the minimum standard to gain the most health benefit and produce the best results.

Amino Acids: The building blocks of protein. There are 20 amino acids used to construct proteins. They have a stimulatory effect on glucagon secretion and a slight effect on insulin. The nine essential amino acids cannot be made by the body and must be obtained through diet. Eggs contain all nine.

Amylase: These enzymes break down carbohydrates. They are secreted by the salivary glands and the pancreas.

Antioxidants: These play a major role in protecting the body from harmful free radicals, which are destructive natural by-products of the body's daily metabolism. Free radicals can also be caused by pollution, smoking and sun. These can lead to premature aging. Examples of antioxidants are Vitamins A, C, and E.

Arachidonic Acid: It is a fatty acid found in all meats, especially red meats and organ meats, and in egg yolks. Some people are very sensitive to this type of fatty acid and have adverse symptoms from consuming those foods. Fish oil can counter some of the effects. It is a precursor to the formation of the bad eicosanoids.

ATP (adenosine triphosphate): It is the basic energy component of the human cell and the main fuel of muscle. It is used during resistance training and lasts less than 20 seconds. To develop *strength*, 45-60 seconds of rest are required between sets. This allows enough of this fuel to be replenished for improved strength.

B Vitamins: It is a complex of some 11 known vitamin factors. They aide in the metabolism of carbohydrates, fats and proteins, to produce vital energy for the body and are water soluble. They are essential for the health of skin, hair, eyes, mouth and liver. They also contribute to the health of the nervous system.

Basal Metabolic Rate BMR: The energy you consume when you are awake but not using any calories to move. It reflects the work your body does to sustain life. This can be increased by 15 percent or more by building muscle and becoming more active.

Beta Cells: These are specialized cells in the pancreas responsible for the production and secretion of insulin.

Beta-Endorphins: Powerful brain chemicals that acts as natural pain killers (the body's morphine pump).

Body Fat Percentage: This is a measure of body composition. It can be obtained by measuring skin fold thickness with calipers, hydrostatic weighing or electrical impedance, the last one being seen frequently in scales and hand held devices. It helps determine your level of body fat which can be an indicator for many diseases and health problems.

Body Mass Index: Is a calculation of body mass based on age, height and weight. It uses a formula to determine the number. The number is used as a way to track trends in a person's overall size. The numbers fall into categories meant to show people at risk for health problems due to their body mass. It is not a failsafe method. Individuals who have a large muscle mass due to weight lifting or genetics might have a false high number although they are very fit.

Body Shape: Genetically determined shape your body would be at its ideal weight. It is due to the way your body stores excess weight in specific areas and not others. It is also determined by your skeletal structure. Shapes are often categorized as "apple," "ruler," "hourglass," "pear," and "inverted triangle." A healthy and fit form can minimize the appearance of these types but they cannot be totally altered by diet or exercise.

CART: Leads the satiety chemicals in the brain and stimulates the hypothalamus to increase metabolism, reduce appetite and increase insulin to deliver energy to muscle cells rather than to be stored as fat.

CCK: A peptide produced in the gastrointestinal track that is released when your bowel senses fat. It delivers a short-term, intense and direct message that indicates fullness.

Calcium: An important mineral that works in conjunction with magnesium to promote bone health, nerve health and muscle building.

Calisthenics Exercise: Part of a vigorous work-out that emphasizes specific muscular work and utilizes resistance.

Carbohydrates–Favorable or High Density: Carbohydrates that break down slowly. This allows a steady release of blood sugar into the bloodstream and results in a low insulin response. Favorable carbohydrates would include most vegetables, certain fruits, and some grains. These foods contain low sugar content or glycemic value. (A.K.A. Complex)

Carbohydrate Sensitivity: A condition faced by some people when eating carbohydrates. They maintain higher insulin levels which is triggered by eating carbohydrates or sugars. This causes intense food cravings and a lack of feeling full. The cause of this condition is unknown but is thought to have genetic and behavioral components.

Carbohydrates–Unfavorable or Low Density: Carbohydrates that are easily digested and break down rapidly. This causes a rapid rise in blood sugar levels and results in a high and rapid insulin response. These are primarily sugars. They are an ideal source of energy, but they enter the blood stream rapidly and are therefore not good for appetite control and blood glucose control. (A.K.A. Simple Sugars)

Chelation: (kee-lay-shun) A process that allows the stomach lining to better absorb minerals. The mineral ion is wrapped in a jacket of amino acids, the building blocks of protein. The stomach then accepts them as if they were protein. This allows for more efficient and complete digestion. Chelated supplements have become popular for their absorption benefits.

Chromium: Mineral that helps maintain proper insulin function. Sufficient amounts can help you build lean muscle and burn fat more efficiently through interaction with the thyroid system. A deficiency stimulates sugary cravings which can create an unhealthy cycle of eating.

Coenzyme Q10: It is responsible for energy conversion. It converts glucose (sugar) to ATP, the energy that powers your cellular functions. It has been shown to improve muscular performance and can help protect muscles from oxidative stress. This can be taken in supplement form.

Complex Carbohydrates: Foods such as whole grains take longer to digest. They break down into glucose or sugar more slowly. Because the body has longer to process them, they are less likely that to be converted into fat. These foods also aid digestion and promote bowel regulation. Sources of complex carbohydrates include grains, beans, fruits and vegetables, and some cereals and pasta.

Cool Down: Slow movements done to lower the heart rate after exercise.

Cortisol: Hormone secreted by adrenal glands in response to stress. It causes a negative chain of events in the body when excess cortisol is present due to chronic stress—things like triggering abdominal fat storage, reduced insulin sensitivity, increased appetite, and it can start a cycle of stress induced eating. No wonder stress control is so important!

Creatine: A naturally occurring amino acid that is found in the body. The majority of creatine (about 95 percent) is located in the skeletal muscle system, and the remaining 5 percent is in the brain, heart and testes. We acquire most of the creatine in our system by consuming meats and fish as well as dairy products, egg whites, nuts and seeds. Creatine's main benefit is its ability to aid in the production of energy. When ATP loses one of its phosphate molecules and becomes ADP (adenosine diphosphate), it must be converted back to ATP. The creatine in our body is mostly stored as creatine phosphate and it will donate its phosphate to the ADP which renews the ATP molecule and it can now produce energy.

Cyclical Exercise: Involves doing short, less than one minute bursts of all out effort. This is followed by easy recovery movement for one to five minutes or until your heart rate recovers, then repeating that pattern.

Dopamine: Dopamine is a neurotransmitter involved in controlling movement, sleep, emotional response, alertness, and addictive behavior. As a chemical messenger, dopamine is similar to adrenaline. It acts as a reward center in the brain and is also involved with the ability to experience pleasure and pain. A number of psychiatric and mood disorders, are attributed to imbalances in dopamine levels. Elevation of dopamine levels often leads to an improvement in mood, alertness, and sex drive. Several nutrients are thought to elevate dopamine levels, including the amino acid tyrosine, and certain B vitamins, such as NADH (the activated form of vitamin B-3, or niacin).

Eicosanoids: A group of hormones that are derived from essential fatty acids, the best known of which are prostaglandins. They are compounds composed of twenty carbon atoms. They are produced in the cells, act inside the cells, vanish in fractions of seconds and regulate the internal equilibrium of each cell. They control and direct many diverse functions in the body. They fall into two groups that have opposing functions.

Endocrine Glands: Ductless glands that empty their secretions directly into the blood stream. The secretions contain specific hormones that influence growth and reproduction.

Energy Balance: How much food energy you *burn* compared to how much you *consume*. Small but consistent imbalances of just fifty calories a day can add or subtract five pounds in a year. Eating too much or moving too little can cause the *storage* of those calories, not burned immediately, in the form of *fat*.

Enriched: Often foods are "enriched" to improve flavor and texture but it decreases the nutritional value of the food. Manufacturers strip the food of its natural healthy properties (often which are not as tasty) and replace them with a list of things they think consumers desire, things that also enhance taste and preserve the product longer.

Enzyme: A protein catalyst that stimulates and accelerates the velocity of chemical changes in the body.

Essential Fatty Acids: Fatty acids that the body needs but cannot make. They must be obtained through diet. They are the building blocks of eicosanoids. They fall into two groups, Omega-6 and Omega-3. Each has its own unique properties.

Fat: It has many positive functions such as providing energy reserves and cushioning our organs and bones. It acts as insulation and it synthesizes estrogen and other hormones. However, it is calorie dense and whatever the body cannot not process immediately will be stored as fat. In the body it gets broken down into smaller pieces and is absorbed as fat. Good fats decrease your body's inflammatory response and bad fats increase it.

Muscles can use fat stored for energy when it has used up all the available carbohydrates.

Flexibility: The body's ability to move through a wide range of motion. Tight muscles lead to lack of flexibility and can increase your chance of injury when performing exercise or routine tasks.

Free Fatty Acid: This is the structural component of fat.

Fructose: A simple sugar found in *fruits*. The insulin stimulating effect is lower than that of galactose and glucose.

Functional Strength: The combination of basic strength abilities plus your coordination at applying that quality at a particular time. It is pivotal in improving balance and mobility.

GABA: Gamma-aminobutyric acid (GABA) is an important inhibitory neurotransmitter in the brain. Excitation in the brain must be balanced with inhibition. Too much excitation can lead to restlessness, irritability, insomnia, and even seizures. GABA is able to induce relaxation, analgesia, and sleep. Barbiturates and benzodiazepines are prescriptions known to stimulate GABA receptors, and bring on relaxation.

Galactose: A simple sugar found in *dairy* products. The insulin stimulating effect is less than glucose.

Ghrelin: Hormone secreted by the stomach that sends hunger signals to the brain twice an hour, three times an hour when very hungry or dieting. This accounts for short-term hunger. As the stomach fills, these levels reduce as does the appetite.

Glucose: A simple sugar in a form that circulates in the bloodstream. It is the body's main energy source. Other sugars are converted into glucose by enzymes before they can be used as an energy source.

Glucagon: The hormone that is the regulatory counterpart of insulin. It is stimulated by dietary protein. It releases stored carbohydrates from the liver to maintain blood sugar at optimal mental performance levels and it helps to metabolize stored fat.

GLUT-4 and Lipoprotein Lipase: Exercise increases these two enzymes. They transport glucose and fat into muscles. Because of these enzymes, after a 60-minute workout, the calories in sugar and fat are more likely to be diverted into *muscle* instead of *fat* tissues.

Glycemic Index: A measure of how rapidly the carbohydrates in food are broken down and turned into sugar in the blood. Also how much it causes blood sugar to rise.

Heme Iron: The iron in red meat. It is bound to protein, a form that the gastrointestinal tract can absorb more easily and completely.

Hemoglobin: Oxygen-carrying protein of red blood cells. This level is evaluated when checking for anemia

High-Density Lipoproteins (HDL) Cholesterol: They return unused fat to the liver for disposal. The levels are raised by aerobic exercise. They are beneficial due their removal effect on the harmful lipoproteins. (A.K.A. Good Cholesterol)

Hormone: A chemical agent secreted by the endocrine glands. They regulate many body functions, including growth, digestion, and fluid balance. Each affects a specific organ and elicits a specific response.

Hypothalamus: Area in the brain that secretes hunger and satiety chemicals. These chemicals cause the push-pull people feel within the hunger and fullness cycle. These are stimulated by the type of foods, how much and how often we eat. They can be manipulated positively or negatively based on our choices.

Insulin: Hormone secreted by the pancreas in response to carbohydrates and to some extent protein. It drives nutrients into the cells for storage. It is most known for its effect on blood sugar regulation.

Insulin Resistance: A condition in which the cells of the body become resistant to the effects of insulin. The normal response to a given amount of insulin is reduced. As a result, higher levels of insulin are needed in order for insulin to have its effects.

Interval Walking: Check pulse while walking and take note of it. Add in a short 10-30 second "sprint" followed by slower recovery walking. Gradually build back to a brisk walk and recheck heart rate. When heart rate recovers, sprint again. Following this pattern regularly will maintain the elevated heart rate even when returning to the slower pace.

Isometric: Static movement. A muscle contraction in which the tension increases, but the muscle length remains the same.

Leptin: A protein secreted by stored fat that reduces appetite and promotes a feeling of fullness and satisfaction in the long term.

Lipase: An enzyme secreted by the pancreas that helps digest fats.

Lipid: A fat of plant or animal origin.

Lipoproteins: They function as the major carrier of lipids and are a combination of fat and proteins that circulate in the bloodstream.

Liver: Acts as the body's metabolic computer. It is an internal organ that directs the metabolism of macronutrients and the manufacture of enzymes, cholesterol, and other important substances.

Low-Density Lipoproteins (LDL) Cholesterol: It is manufactured in the liver and circulates throughout the body. It is known for making its fat available to all body cells and is thought to be a major risk factor for heart disease. (A.K.A. Bad Cholesterol)

Lymphatic System: The main route of absorption for fats from the small intestine. They are small vessels that drain tissue fluid back into the cardiovascular system.

Macronutrients: They are protein, carbohydrates and fat. Only macronutrients have any effect on hormone secretion.

Magnesium: An important mineral that works in conjunction with calcium to promote bone health, nerve health and muscle building.

Maltose: A kind of sugar composed of two molecules of glucose. It is formed by the hydrolysis of starch and is converted into glucose by the enzyme maltase.

Melatonin: It a hormone produced in the pineal gland, a small gland in the brain, which helps regulate sleep and wake cycles. Very small amounts of melatonin are found in foods such as meats, grains, fruits, and vegetables. It is also available as a dietary supplement used to treat jet lag or sleep problems (insomnia). Natural melatonin production is partly affected by light. During the shorter days of the winter months, melatonin production may start earlier or, more often, later. This change can lead to symptoms of seasonal affective disorder (SAD), or winter depression. Natural melatonin levels decline gradually with age.

Metabolism: The rate at which your body burns calories for fuel. Influenced by activity level, genetics, age, medications, body composition, thyroid function and the amount of *lean muscle* you have. The more muscle mass you have, the higher your metabolism will be. Just one pound of muscle burns 35 to 50 more calories per day!

Micronutrients: They are vitamins and minerals. Micronutrients are used by enzymes in the body and are supplied by the diet or through supplementation. Adequate levels improve the efficiency of the metabolism and body regulation.

Minerals: They are found in food and are vital in the development of strength, fitness and growth of the body. Calcium, phosphorus, iodine and magnesium have specific daily requirements. Other essential minerals are potassium and sodium. There are also trace minerals or elements that are known to enhance proper nutrition.

Mitochondria: Calorie burners in muscle cells that create ATP from the energy that we consume. In the cell compartment, they burn fat and sugar to fuel and feed muscle fibers and aid in general muscle maintenance.

Monounsaturated fatty acids (MUFAs pronounced MOO-fahs): They are fat molecules that contain only one double bond. These *healthy fats* are found in olives, peanuts and pecans.

Muscle Loss: This happens when people lose too much weight, too fast. By dieting alone, most people lose 25 to 30 percent of non-fat such as water, lean tissue, bone and muscle. The faster they lose, the less of what is lost comes from fat.

Muscle Power: The ability to move as rapidly as possible or to overcome a resistance in the shortest possible time.

Muscle Response: Increased muscle tone occurs as a response to stress put on the muscle. It causes small tears in the muscle fibers. It is the repair of these small tears that will increase the tone and muscle fibers themselves. This occurs with sufficient rest and nutrition.

Muscle Strength: The ability to produce maximal force regardless of the duration involved in doing so.

Muscular Endurance: The ability to perform less than an all-out effort for an extended period of time.

Norepinephrine: The amino acids phenylalanine and tyrosine are converted into dopamine, which, in turn, is converted into norepinephrine. Increases in brain levels of norepinephrine lead to arousal and mood elevation, but excessive amounts can cause irritability, anxiety, and insomnia.

NPY: A protein called neuropeptide Y that drives the eating chemicals, which have the opposite effect of CART on the hypothalamus; it decreases metabolism and increases appetite.

Nutrients: Quality in food that your body uses for a specific purpose. Each is used differently by the body and processed in unique ways.

Nutritional Supplements: Pills, powders or liquids containing vitamins, minerals, nutrients or enzymes. They are designed to make up for deficits in nutritional intake. Can be used in coordination with a proper diet to enhance optimum health and body functioning.

Omega-3 Fatty Acids: Improves immune and cardiovascular function and includes essential long-chain fatty acids such as DHA and EPA. ALA, a short-chain fatty acid, must be metabolized to a long chain fatty acid for significant impact. Increased consumption has health benefits.

Omega-6 Fatty Acids: They are the building blocks for both "good" and "bad" types of eicosanoids. An excess can lead to the build up of the "bad" eicosanoids. An increase in Omega-3 fatty acids can inhibit the production of the "bad" type.

Osteoporosis: The loss of bone mass that can lead to brittle and weak bones, prone to fracture.

Pancreas: An elongated, narrow organ about the length of your hand. It is located behind the stomach and plays an essential roll in controlling the fuel that is made available to the cells of the body. It does this through the release of three hormones—insulin, glucagon and somatostatin.

Phytates: Iron from green leafy vegetables is bound to this compound. The human intestine does not readily digest this.

Polyunsaturated Fats: These are fat molecules that contain two or more double bonds. This includes most vegetable oils.

Potassium: An important mineral for maintaining body functions. It has a role in the passage of nerve impulses, muscle contraction and the maintenance of blood pressure. A deficiency can result from a rapid loss of fluid. This can be from vomiting, diarrhea, excess sweating or a radical diet change.

Probiotics: These are dietary supplements or foods that contain beneficial, bacteria that are similar to those normally found in your body. These microorganisms may provide some of the same health benefits that the bacteria already existing in your body do—such as assisting with digestion and helping protect against harmful bacteria.

Proper Form: Each exercise is designed to work specific muscle groups. Proper form denotes that you are able to maintain the correct body positioning that will work the muscle in both the contraction and extension phases of the movement. Failure to do so will result in lack of desired definition and possible injury. It is an essential component.

Protein: A nutrient that can be found in meat, eggs, beans, and dairy. Proteins are broken down into small amino acids, which then go to the liver. If they are not needed for muscle growth or maintenance, they will get converted to glucose (sugar), which will then be converted to fat if you don't use it for energy. It is necessary for red blood cell formation, muscle growth and maintenance. It decreases appetite by stabilizing blood sugar and promoting fullness.

Push-Pull Phenomenon: This is what happens when you diet. Your body fights to release fat while, at the same time, your fat cells are constantly striving to fill themselves up with *more* fat. Your body perceives dieting as gradual starvation. Traditional dieting involves you deliberately withholding the body's usual supply of nutrients and energy sources. The body will attempt to fight off this potentially dangerous depletion of energy stores by *slowing down your metabolism* and you may experience this as a weight loss slow down or plateau.

Recovery Heart Rate: Your heart rate taken at the end of activity after a stretch or cool down. It is used to gauge when the heart rate has returned to the pre-exercise pulse.

Rep. or Repetition: One complete movement from start to finish.

Repetition Maximum RM: A 12 RM weight is a weight with which a person could perform 12 movements or reps in *proper form*. Shown to increase lean muscle mass. Six or fewer reps with greater weight will result in more muscle power with less mass. Fifteen plus RM will build muscle endurance with only minor strength gains.

Resistance Training: The purposeful contraction of muscles through exercise for the purpose of building strength, endurance and/or tone. Builds lean muscle mass which boosts metabolism and energy. Supports the behavior changes needed for success and life long weight management. This includes calisthenics, weight training and isometrics.

Resting Heart Rate: It is an average of your heart rate when doing no activity. Usually taken in the morning before getting out of bed for several days and averaged.

Ribose: Ribose is fundamental to the existence of all living cells and functions as the sole regulator in the production of ATP (adenosine-triphosphate), the most basic source of all cellular energy. It is the carbohydrate backbone of genetic material and is also core to the production of many essential metabolic compounds. Ribose aids the body to produce cellular energy in low oxygen conditions more efficiently, allowing the body more energy for recovery, delivery of nutrients, and growth and repair of tissues. It has been used off-label to aid low energy conditions.

Sarcopenia: The loss of muscle mass, strength and function that occur per decade, after age 40. It is thought that without exercise and a healthy diet, there is a loss of 3 percent to 5 percent of muscle mass—per decade.

Saturated Fats: These are fat molecules that contain carbon atoms fully bound with hydrogen atoms. They are found in most animal fats.

Selenium: A mineral anti-oxidant that works with Vitamin E to produce the body's own natural free-radical fighter, glutathione. It promotes a healthy immune system and has anti-aging properties. A deficiency could contribute to elevated cholesterol.

Serotonin: Serotonin is a neurotransmitter, which is a type of chemical that sends messages back and forth in the brain. These brain chemicals are thought to influence feelings of hunger and fullness. Serotonin helps regulate a wide range of psychological and biological functions including mood, anxiety, arousal, and aggression. Many antidepressant medications are targeted to elevate serotonin levels.

Set: One series of RM. Frequently one to three sets are performed. This is determined based on desired goal and fitness level. One set of 10 RM is a good goal for beginners.

Set Point: The weight at which your body struggles to remain, regardless of the outside pressures on it to change. The body is designed to keep you healthy and protect you from starvation. The closer you get to your goal weight the more your body is going to cling to what is already there.

Simple Sugars: These are carbohydrates that are easily digested and that rapidly increase blood sugar levels. When sugar is quickly absorbed and sent to the liver for digestion, it tells your body to turn that sugar into fat if it cannot be used immediately for energy. When consumed, they cause a short-term and temporary energy boost, which is followed by a rebounding effect that causes you to crave more to recreate the effect, causing an energy spike and crash cycle.

Steady State Metabolism: What your body switches to after 20 minutes of sustained exercise. During this time changes occur that positively influence the body's ability to function aerobically (20 minutes and beyond creates increased calorie burning potential and the **most overall benefits—Super-burn!**).

Stretching: A static body pose that is performed by bending or extending the body or body part and holding that position in order to stretch muscles. This is an important fitness component.

Target Heart Rate: It is a percentage of exertion measured by taking your heart rate during exercise. It is based on your age and your pulse. It can help you determine the intensity of your effort.

Target Heart Rate Range: Basic formula is 220 minus your age, multiplied by the percentage of intensity (usually between 55 and 85 percent).

Thyroid Function: This gland regulates metabolism by secreting a hormone called thyroxine. *The amount you secrete is influenced by what you eat.* Consume fewer calories than your body burns and your thyroid tries to compensate by cutting back on thyroxine. This causes your metabolism to slow down and you feel sluggish, so you do not move around as much—a self-defeating situation. This is a normal function designed to conserve body tissue during times of famine. Such extremes can cause BMR to plummet. That is another reason to not cut calories too drastically when trying to lose weight. It can backfire and also cause irritability and lack of energy.

Training Effect: It is the physiologic adaptations that occur as a result of aerobic exercise. There must be sufficient intensity, frequency and duration to produce beneficial changes in the body.

Trans Fats: Can be produced by heating oil. They are similar to saturated fats. They increase the LDL or harmful cholesterol and decrease the HDL or beneficial cholesterol. This type of fat should be avoided when possible.

Tryptophan: The starting point in making serotonin is tryptophan, one of the amino acids we ingest through food, particularly meat, fish, and other protein foods. If enough tryptophan is not supplied to the brain, serotonin levels drop. Tryptophan is converted into 5-HTP, which is then converted into serotonin. After serotonin is made, the pineal gland is able to convert it at night into the sleep hormone melatonin.

Vitamins: Components of food that are metabolized by the body for specific functioning. They are used by the body to promote optimal functioning. Can be supplemented, but works more efficiently when obtained through the food.

Vitamins A, D, E and K: These are fat-soluble vitamins that support immune system function and provide antioxidant protection.

Vitamin C: It is involved in immune system health and promotes collagen formation. It is a potent antioxidant, which helps fight free radicals, known to damage cells.

Warm-Up: Slow fluid movements done to prepare muscles for exercise. Helps to prevent injury and promotes flexibility.

Weight Bearing Exercise: Any exercise that puts good *stress* on the bones. Bones constantly adapt to the mechanical stress you put on them, much like muscle. In fact, it is the muscle action pulling on bone that stimulates new bone to grow. So focus on your total body!

Weight Cycling: This is what occurs when rapid weight loss causes reduction in lean muscle. The resulting decreased metabolism causes the body to not burn calories as well as it did before dieting. As a result, eating normally again can cause even more weight gain than you had prior to the diet due to this decrease in metabolism.

Weight Loss Formula: To lose one pound of fat in a week you must decrease your normal calorie intake by 500 calories a day or 3,500 per week. This can be done through diet or a combo of diet and burning calories through exercise (BEST).

Yo-Yo Diets: Restriction diets that cause people to lose weight fast at first but are so restrictive that people will not stick to them long term. This causes *weight cycling* and leads to ongoing issues with body image, weight gain, depression and discouragement.

REFERENCES

American Heart Association, www.americanheart.org

Appleton, N. *Lick the Sugar Habits.* Garden City Park, NY: Avery Publishing Group Inc., 2005.

Bain, D. *Destination Success.* Grand Rapids, MI: Fleming Revel, 2005.

Bourne, E., and L. Garono. *Coping with Anxiety.* Oakland, CA: New Harbinger Publications, Inc., 2003.

Brio, B. *Beyond Success.* Asheville, NC: Pygmalion Press, 1999.

Burns, D. *Feeling Good.* New York: Avon Books/HarperCollins, 1980.

Byrne, R. *The Secret.* New York: Atria Books Simon & Schuster, Inc., 2006.

Canfield, J. *The Success Principles.* New York: HarperCollins, 2005.

Canfield, J., M. Hansen and L. Hewitt. *The Power of FOCUS.* Deerfield Beach, FL: Health Communications Inc., 2000.

Carlson, R. *Don't Sweat the Small Stuff.* New York: Hyperion, 1998.

Carlson, R. *Don't Worry Make Money.* New York: Hyperion, 1997.

Carlson, R. *What About the BIG STUFF?.* New York: Hyperion, 2002.

Cherniski, S. *Caffeine Blues.* New York: Warner Books, 1998.

Centers for Disease Control and Prevention, www.cdc.gov

Chopra, D. *Ageless Body Timeless Mind.* New York: Harmony Books, 1993.

Cloud, H., and J. Townsend. *Boundaries.* Grand Rapids, MI: Zondervan Publishing House, 1992.

Cloud, H., and J. Townsend. *It's Not My Fault.* Nashville, TN: Integrity Publishers, 2007.

Covey, S. *The 7 Habits of Highly Effective People.* New York: A Fireside Book, Simon & Schuster, 1989.

DesMaisons, K. *The Sugar Addict's Total Recovery Program.* New York: Ballantine, 2000.

Eades, M.R, and M.D. Eades. *Protein Power.* New York: Bantam, 1996.

Emotions Anonymous, www.emotionsanonymous.org

Fritz, R. *Fast Track.* Naperville, IL: Inside Advantage, 1999.

Gabriel, J. *The Gabriel Method.* New York: Atria Books, 2008.

Garcia, O. *The Balance.* New York: ReganBooks, 1998.

Gordon, G. *The Omega-3 Miracle.* Topanga, CA: Freedom Press, 2006.

Gray, J. *How to Get What You Want and Want What You Have.* New York: HaperCollins, 1999.

Greene, R., and L. Feldon. *Perfect Balance.* New York: Clarkson Potter, 2005.

Haggi, J. *How to Win Over Worry.* Eugene, OR: Harvest House Publishers, 2001.

Halprin, S. *Winning after Losing.* New York: Hachette Book Group USA, 2007.

Harris, V. *The Productivity Epiphany.* Trenton, Missouri: Beckworth Publications, 2008.

Hart, A. *Adrenalin and Stress.* Waco Texas: Word Books, 1986.

Hay, L. *You Can Heal Your Life.* Carlsbad, CA: Hay House Inc., 2004.

Heller, R., and R. Heller. *The Carbohydrate Addict's Diet.* New York: Signet, 1993.

Hicks, E., and J. Hicks. *The Amazing Power of Deliberate Intent.* Carlsbad, CA: Hay House, 2006.

Hoeger, W., and S. Hoeger. *Lifetime Physical Fitness & Wellness.* Belmont, CA: Thomson Wadsworth, 2007.

Holt, S. *Combat Syndrome X, Y and Z.* Paterson, NJ: Wellness Publishing, 2002.

Jordan, M. *Fitness Theroy & Practice.* California: Aerobics and Fitness Association of America, and Reebok University Press, 1997.

Karas, J. *Flip the Switch.* New York: Three Rivers Press, 2002.

Kowalski, R. *The 8-Week Cholesterol Cure.* New York: HarperTorch, 2002.

Lena, D., and M. Lena. *Being Better Than Your Best.* Chicago, IL: Possibility Press, 2003.

Kushner, H. *When All You've Ever Wanted Isn't Enough.* New York: Pocket Books Simon & Schuster Inc., 1986.

Littauer, F. *Personality Plus.* Grand Rapids MI: Baker Book House Company, 1994.

Lorig, K., Holman, H., Sobel, D., Laurent, D., Gonzalez, V., and M. Minor. *Living A Healthy Life With Chronic Conditions.* Boulder, CO: Bull Publishing Company, 2006.

Markova, D. *I Will Not Die an Unlived Life.* San Francisco, CA: Conari Press, 2000.

Mayo Clinic, www.mayoclinic.com

McMeekin, G. *The 12 Secrets of Highly Creative Women.* New York: MJF Books, 2000.

Meyer, J. *Battlefield of the Mind.* Tulsa, OK: Harrison House, 1995.

Meyer, J. *Be Anxious for Nothing.* Tulsa, OK: Harrison House, 1998.

Meyer, J. *Eat and Stay Thin.* Tulsa, OK: Harrison House, 1999.

Meyer, J. *How to Succeed at Being Yourself.* Tulsa, OK: Harrison House, 1999.

Meyer, J. *I Dare You.* New York: Hachette Book Group USA, 2007.

Meyer, J. *Look Great Feel Great.* New York: Warner Faith, 2006.

Meyer, J. *Never Give Up.* New York: Hachette Book Group USA, 2008.

Meyer, J. *Secrets to Exceptional Living.* Tulsa, OK: Harrison House, 2002.

Meyer, J. *The Power of Being Positive.* New York: Warner Faith, 2003.

Moore, J. *Seizing the Moments.* Nashville, TN: Abingdon Press, 1988.

Osteen, J. *Become A Better You.* New York: Free Press, 2008.

Osteen, J. *Your Best Life Now.* New York: Warner Faith, 2004.

Peale , N. *Power of the Plus Factor.* Old Tappan, NJ: Fleming H. Revell Company, 1987.

Peale, N. *Reaching Your Potential.* New York: Wings Books, 1990.

Peale, N. *Staying Alive All Your Life.* Pawling, NY: Simon & Schuster, 1997

Peale, N. *How To Make Positive Imaging Work For You.* Old Tappan, NJ: Fleming H. Revell Company, 1982.

Sarino, J. *Healing Back Pain.* New York: Warner Books, 1991.

Sears, B. and B. Lawren. *The Zone.* New York: HarperCollins, 1995.

Schuller, R. *If It's Going To Be It's Up To Me.* San Francisco, CA: HarperSanFrancisco, 1997.

Shaevitz, M. *The Confident Woman.* New York: Harmony Books, 1999.

Simpson LeSourd, S. *The Compulsive Woman.* Grand Rapids, MI: Fleming H. Revell, 1987.

St. James, E. *Simplify Your Life.* New York: Hyperion, 1994.

Roizen, M. and M. Oz. *You Being Beautiful.* New York: Free Press, 2008.

Roizen, M. and M. Oz. *You On A Diet.* New York: Free Press, 2006.

Ruggiero, V. *Good Habits.* Louisville, KY: Westminster/John Knox Press, 1991.

Savard, M. and C. Svec. *The Body Shape Solution to Weight Loss and Wellness.* New York: Atria Books, 2005.

Smith, H. *The 10 Natural Laws of Successful Time And Life Management.* New York: Time Warner, 1994.

Statman, P. *Life On A Balance Beam.* Oakland, CA: Piccolo Press, 1998.

Superko, R. and L. Tucker. *Before the Heart Attacks.* United States Of Americal: Rodale, 2003.

Tolle, E. *The Power of Now.* Novato, CA: New World Library, 1999.

Tracy, B. *Eat That Frog!* Naperville, IL: Simple Truths, 2008.

United States Department of Agriculture, www.mypyramid.gov

Vaccariello, L. *Flat Belly Diet.* New York: Rodale Inc., 2008.

Weber, B. *Conquering the Kill-Joys.* Waco, TX: Word Books, 1986.

Warren, R. *The Purpose Driven Life.* Grand Rapids, MI: Zondervan Publishing House, 2002.

Waterhouse, D. *Outsmarting The Female Fat Cell.* New York: Warner Books, 1993.

Weil, A. *8 Weeks To Optimum Health.* New York: Alfred A. Knopf, 2006.

Weil, A. *Healthy Aging.* New York: Alfred A. Knopf, 2005.

Whitt, J. *Road Signs for Success.* Broken Arrow, OK: Dream House Publishers, 2002.

Williams, S. *Essentials of Nutrition and Diet Therapy.* St. Louis: Mosby, 1994.

Helpful Tools

Internet: It is full of information, almost *too* much! Some of the information even contradicts itself. Sometimes I wonder, "Where did this information really come from? Can I really trust it?" It is easy to become overwhelmed and not utilize the valuable tools that it can provide. Use the Internet wisely and check the sources of the information.

Make sure they are not trying to sell you something or have hidden interests in shading the information. Website addresses that end in .gov indicate a government site and can usually be noted as credible sources. Never trust Wikipedia, the online encyclopedia. It is built and edited by users and can be altered incorrectly.

Library: Don't forget about the numerous resources at the library. Besides books, they have free Internet access and people there to help you. The health and wellness related topics are numerous. Many books, magazines or guides will show examples and give sample exercise plans. There is a style and format to fit everyone's needs. All you have to do is look.

Find a book to read for **pleasure** as well. As you feed your mind with info, you can feed your spirit with some relaxing activity. It can be a time to rediscover a favorite genre or author. Once you find a new style that intrigues you, time will fly and relaxation will overtake you! This may take some trial and error to discover. Have fun exploring.

Regularly choose some motivational books to encourage and uplift you. Like any type of book, you may have to try different authors and styles before you find one that is beneficial to you. This can improve your mental outlook and attitude.

Try taking the kids to get some children's books as well. Reinforce their love of reading by modeling and encouraging the behavior. The library also has a wide range of videos and audio books. If you have not been to the library in a while, check it out! (Pun intended)

Audio Books and Videos: Take a look at the audio-visual media available. Audio books are great for getting out and walking. They help the time to fly and keep you going to find out what will happen next. The laps fly by when you get hooked into a story.

It is also good for commuters who spend more time on the road than they do sitting and reading. You can *experience* a story without turning pages. Mixing it up with different videos or audio books can keep things new. Downloading podcasts to your MP3 player can also be a fun option.

With current technology, the possibilities are endless! Exercise does not have to be a drain on your time. It can become a time of restoration when you create things to look forward to—like listening to the latest audio book from your favorite author.

Parks and Trails: Check out the parks and trails offered in your area. Often people overlook the obvious. Walking and hiking trails are wonderful ways to change up your fitness routine. It is important to locate outdoor fitness opportunities. They allow you to experience the outdoors, an important component of wellness, as you exercise. Look for fairs and festivals in your area, to see if they are offering any walk/run competitions. These types of offerings will give you an event to train for and can be extremely motivating.

Local Gym or Fitness Center: Make a point to stop in at a gym or fitness center. Most will have a trainer on duty that can help you establish an exercise program. A few visits with a professional can pay big dividends in your progress. Learning proper form and technique can make vast improvements in your overall results.

This is another place to obtain free resources. If they have a reading area with magazines or fitness books, you can get some quick inspiration and direction. Enrolling in a new fitness class can spark your imagination, while at the same time teaching you new moves for your personal routine. It is a great way to add some life to a general fitness plan.

It is always wise to be around people who have similar fitness goals. They help to keep you on track and can provide inspiration. You could find a workout partner or even an encouraging new friend. Having these kinds of support people around will help you stick to your goals. Putting yourself in a healthy environment will not only influence your routine, but also your outlook.

Worthwhile Websites

To create an online fitness calendar:

- www.bam.gov/sub_physicalactivity/cal_index.asp

Credible Health-Related Resources:

- Centers for Disease Control and Prevention: www.cdc.gov
- American Heart Association: www.americanheart.org

Need help analyzing food choices and guidance to make better ones? Utilize the many tools to track, log and evaluate food and activity.

- www.mypyramid.gov
- www.sparkpeople.com
- www.shapefit.com

To find group support:

- Bible-based weight loss group: www.firstplace.org
- Weight loss support group: www.weightwatchers.org
- For daily inspiration and motivation: www.walkthetalk.com

For actual exercises explained and in motion. It is easy to use and free!

- www.thetrainingstationinc.com
- www.sparkpeople.com

Want to know how many calories you are burning with activity?

- www.caloriesperhour.com
- www.nutristrategy.com/activitylist3.htm

Want to know how far you are walking or running? Check out this site:

- www.mapmywalk.com

Want to learn more about sugar sensitivity? This is a great resource to learn more about it and the brain chemicals involved.

- www.radiantrecovery.com

To find out your REAL health age, based on how you live:

- www.realage.com

To find out calorie needs based on your goals, take this assessment:

- www.docmagi.com/Assessment.htm

ABOUT THE AUTHOR

Lisa Stottlemyre Schilling is a wife and mother of three boys. She lives in rural Missouri and embraces the joys and woes of small town living. Lisa uses her enthusiasm for health and fitness promotion to create wellness opportunities for adults, children and organizations.

This endeavor comes from the belief that God blesses people, so they may be a blessing to others. Working through many of life's challenges has taught her to appreciate and value *everyday life*. She feels passionate about sharing this knowledge and her time to empower others to improve their personal health and wellness. As an outspoken advocate for wellness and prevention, her motto is: *"See one, do one, teach one!"*

If you would like to have Lisa Schilling speak to your group about any of the topics covered or you would like to begin a *Personal Accountability Program* you may call 660-654-2548 or contact the Trenton Area Chamber of Commerce (660-359-4324) for more information. You may also check out her website www.getrealwellnesssolutions.com or e-mail her at getrealwellnesssolutions@yahoo.com.

Lisa uses a no-nonsense approach to guide the reader. She offers 20 "Get REAL" Concepts to help you reframe your thinking for this task and five concrete steps to create your own Personal Wellness Plan.

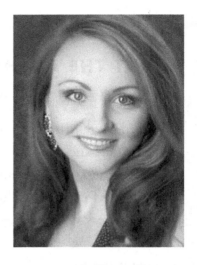

She helps you use what you have to create what you hope for. This guide includes everything you will need to create a flexible personal plan based on your own unique style, natural inclinations and time demands.

It provides a flexible reference for long-term success. She will guide you to create an outline that allows you to fill in the pieces. This means you can bend and not break when life throws you a curve. Let's face it, in REAL life there is distraction, deviation, and the unexpected.

You need a REAL lifestyle plan that you can apply to any situation. This guide was created for people who have struggled with weight, fitness and health issues and are READY to make a change.

Lisa's friendly and down-to-earth style will keep you turning pages and jotting notes. This is not your typical Wellness Guide. It takes a realistic look at life and the reasons that so many people face challenges in these areas. Remember that your level of commitment to your plan will directly affect its ability to change your life.

So what are you doing still reading the back of this book? Get started—and by the way, congrats on taking the first step to your improved total wellness. I knew you could do it!